# ISLAMIC BIOETHICS

Current Issues & Challenges

# Intercultural Dialogue in Bioethics

**Series Editor:** Alireza Bagheri
*(Tehran University of Medical Sciences, Iran)*

---

*Published*

Vol. 1   Islamic Perspectives on the Principles of Biomedical Ethics
*edited by Mohammed Ghaly (Hamad Bin Khalifa University, Qatar)*

Vol. 2   Islamic Bioethics: Current Issues and Challenges
*by Alireza Bagheri (Tehran University of Medical Sciences, Iran) and
Khalid Alali (Qatar University, Qatar)*

*Forthcoming*

Indigenous Bioethics: Local and Global Perspectives
*edited by Linda Briskman (Western Sydney University, Australia),
Deborah Zion (Victoria University, Australia) and
Alireza Bagheri (Tehran University of Medical Sciences, Iran)*

■ Intercultural Dialogue in Bioethics — Vol. 2

Series Editor: Alireza Bagheri

# ISLAMIC BIOETHICS

## Current Issues & Challenges

editors

**Alireza Bagheri**

Tehran University of Medical Sciences, Iran

**Khalid Alali**

Qatar University, Qatar

W**♦ World Scientific**

EW JERSEY · LONDON · SINGAPORE · BEIJING · SHANGHAI · HONG KONG · TAIPEI · CHENNAI · TOKYO

*Published by*

World Scientific Publishing Europe Ltd.

57 Shelton Street, Covent Garden, London WC2H 9HE

*Head office:* 5 Toh Tuck Link, Singapore 596224

*USA office:* 27 Warren Street, Suite 401-402, Hackensack, NJ 07601

**Library of Congress Cataloging-in-Publication Data**

Names: Bagheri, Alireza, editor. | Alali, Khalid, editor.
Title: Islamic bioethics : current issues and challenges / edited by
  Alireza Bagheri, Khalid Alali.
Other titles: Islamic bioethics (Bagheri) | Intercultural dialogue in bioethics ; vol. 2.
Description: New Jersey : World Scientific, 2017. | Series: Intercultural dialogue in bioethics ;
  volume 2 | Includes bibliographical references and index.
Identifiers: LCCN 2017026739 | ISBN 9781783267491 (hardcover : alk. paper)
Subjects: | MESH: Bioethical Issues | Islam | Ethics, Medical | Religion and Medicine
Classification: LCC R725.59 | NLM WB 60 | DDC 174.20917/67--dc23
LC record available at https://lccn.loc.gov/2017026739

**British Library Cataloguing-in-Publication Data**
A catalogue record for this book is available from the British Library.

Printed in Singapore

# Contents

# Contributors

**Khalid Alali** is Professor of Human Genetics in the Department of Biological Science and the Director of the Foundation Program of Qatar University. He was the Chairperson of the UNESCO World Commission on the Ethics of Scientific and Technology (COMEST).

**Mohammad Ali Albar** is the Director of Medical Ethics Center in the International Medical Center in Jeddah, Saudi Arabia. He is a Counselor to The International Islamic Fiqh Academy as well as the Islamic Fiqh Council.

**Alireza Bagheri** is Assistant Professor of Medicine and Medical Ethics, Tehran University of Medical Sciences. He is a member of the UNESCO International Bioethics Committee (IBC) and an elected Fellow of The Hastings Center, New York.

**Azizan Baharuddin** is Professor and the Director of the Institute of Islamic Understanding in Malaysia. She is a member of the UNESCO International Bioethics Committee and a member of the Drafting Committee of the International Islamic Declaration on Climate Change.

**Alastair Campbell** is Professor of Medical Ethics and Emeritus Director of the Center for Biomedical Ethics in National University of Singapore. He is an elected Fellow of The Hastings Center, and a member of the Bioethics Advisory Committee to the Singapore Government.

**Hassan Chamsi-Pasha** is Professor and the Head of Non-Invasive Cardiology in King Fahd Armed Forces Hospital, Jeddah, Saudi Arabia. He is a Counselor to The International Islamic Fiqh Academy.

**Jonathan Crane** is Professor of Bioethics and Jewish Thought at Emory University's Center for Ethics, USA. He is the founder and co–editor-in-chief of the Journal of Jewish Ethics.

**Abdallah Daar** is Professor of Public Health Sciences at the Dalla Lana Faculty of Public Health, University of Toronto. He is a laureate of the UNESCO Avicenna Prize for Ethics of Science and an elected Fellow of The Hastings Center, New York.

**Abul Fadl Mohsin Ebrahim** is Emeritus Professor of Islamic Studies at the School of Religion, University of KwaZulu-Natal, South Africa. He specializes in Islamic history, law, ethics, theology, and bioethics and has written extensively in these fields.

**Hakan Ertin** is a Professor in the Department of History of Medicine and Ethics, Faculty of Medicine, Istanbul University, Turkey.

**Nazafarin Ghasemzadeh** is a PhD candidate in medical ethics in Tehran University of Medical Sciences. She teaches medical ethics at Urmia University of Medical Sciences, Iran.

**Ilhan Ilkilic** is a Professor in the Department of History of Medicine and Ethics, Faculty of Medicine, Istanbul University, Turkey.

**Bagher Larijani** is Professor of Endocrinology and Internal Medicine and Director of the Endocrinology and Metabolism Research Center, Iran. He is the Head of Medical Ethics and History of Medicine Research Center in the Tehran University of Medical Sciences.

**Mansoureh Madani** is a PhD candidate in medical ethics, Tehran University of Medical Sciences. She studied Islamic Philosophy (MA) and Theology (BA) and teaches medical ethics in Qom University, Iran.

**Ingrid Mattson** is Professor of Islamic Studies at Huron University College at Western University, Canada. She served as Vice-President, then as President of the Islamic Society of North America (USA), the first woman to serve in either position.

**Mohd Noor Musa** is a Research Officer at the Institute of Islamic Understanding and an affiliate member of the National Bioethics Council in Malaysia. He is a member of a multidisciplinary group of researchers focusing on religion, sustainability and environment.

**Tariq Ramadan** is Professor of Contemporary Islamic Studies in the University of Oxford and is the Director of the Center for Islamic Legislation and Ethics in Doha, Qatar.

**James Rusthoven** is Professor Emeritus, Department of Oncology in McMaster University. He is a bioethicist physician and currently serves as a medical officer in Health Canada where he reviews new biologics for consideration of authorization for the treatment of cancer patients.

**Gamal Serour** is Professor of Obstetrics and Gynaecology and Director of International Islamic Center for Population Studies and Research, Al-Azhar University. He is the Immediate Past President of the International Federation of Gynecology and Obstetrics.

**Mehrunisha Suleman** is a post-doctoral researcher at the Centre of Islamic Studies, University of Cambridge. She holds a medical degree from the University of Oxford and completed her Alimiyyah degree with Al Salaam Institute.

**Carol Taylor** is Professor of Medicine and Nursing in Georgetown University and a founding member and former director of the Pellegrino Center for Clinical Bioethics. She is a Senior Clinical Scholar at the Kennedy Institute of Ethics, USA.

# Preface

While the dialogue between Christian and Jewish bioethics is well established, Islamic bioethics, which has a rich and diverse history of development, adds yet another valuable ethnocentric cultural context to the global discussion.

Ten Have and Gordijn (2014) argue that whatever the precise historic origins of bioethics, currently it has turned into a truly global phenomenon and the interpretation and application of a bioethics framework must always be informed by local circumstances. Sachedina (2012) concurs and emphasizes that the subject matter of bioethics is "an admixture of ethnocentric cultural context connected to geography, history, language, and ethnic tension of each community."

Bioethics is often regarded as a typically western phenomenon first developed in North America, then adopted in Western Europe, and recently exported to other parts of the world (ten Have and Gordijn 2014). However, it has been argued that western bioethics has been imported in other countries without sufficiently taking into account indigenous and traditional value systems (Chattopadhyay 2011). As observed by Brockopp (2008), scholarship on bioethics in Europe and North America often does not connect with ongoing scholarship in the Muslim world and *vice versa*.

As a result, ethicists on both sides underestimate the complexity of the others' positions while at the same time missing many points of possible convergence.

In bioethics literature, there is great interest in religion's role in bioethical discussion and norms. Diverse opinions from religious-based and non–religious-based points of view contribute to a spectrum of recommendations. Defending what has been called "irreligious bioethics," Timothy (2012) posits that "irreligious skepticism toward religious views about health, healthcare practices and institutions, and responses to biomedical innovations can yield important benefits to the field. Irreligious skepticism makes it possible to raise questions that otherwise go unasked and to protect against the overreach of religion." As Alastair Campbell reminds us, global bioethics must respect the whole diversity of world views of ethics, both religious and non-religious (Campbell 1999). In each society, the answer to the following question reflects that society's cultural norms: to what extent should religious norms inform and influence bioethical debates? However, given the multiculturalism as well as the diversity within each society it is hard to imagine that the answer can be an absolute yes or no. Therefore, in today's globalized world, knowledge about religious bioethics, and how it influences behaviour as well as decision making, is important not only for religious societies but also for non-religious societies.

The participation of Islamic bioethics scholars in a dialogue with other religious-based bioethics scholars is crucial. Such a dialogue, with a rigorous examination of comparative religious ethics, would help scholars in the field share their concerns as well as practical solutions for bioethical dilemmas. However as it has been suggested, Islamic bioethics needs to construct a language that is understood across cultures and traditions to take advantage of the opportunity to converse with scholars about other religious or secular bioethics approaches (Sachedina 2012). To initiate conversation with secular or other religion-based bioethicists, Muslim scholars should not only understand the underpinnings of moral deliberations in secular or other religion-based bioethics but also make efforts to share the foundations of the Islamic theological–ethical deliberations.

This volume will contribute significantly to on-going scholarly and public bioethics discourses in the Islamic context. It provides an elucidation of Islamic bioethics, and is also an invitation for Islamic bioethics scholars to become more conversant partners with scholars in other religious and non-religious traditions of ethical reflection. Islamic bioethics refers primarily to Islamic normative pronouncements that appeal to Islamic religious authority. Respect for Islamic religious norms is essential for the legitimacy of bioethical standards in the Muslim context (Ayman Shabana 2013). As observed by Farhat Moazam, in Islamic bioethics, discussions and rulings are not fashioned in a vacuum but shaped by the interplay of perceived boundaries of authority within political and legal systems and existing societal norms (Moazam 2011).

The chapters provide firsthand Islamic perspectives on specific bioethical topics, such as brain death, stem cell research, gender ethics, environmental ethics, and the physician–patient relationship. Furthermore, this book enhances the international understanding of Islamic bioethics in a more comprehensive articulation by presenting broader theological–ethical beliefs.

In chapter one, Tariq Ramadan elaborates on the sources, methodology and application of Islamic ethics. The author emphasizes the importance of studying ethics in relation to law, jurisprudence (*fiqh*), philosophy–theology as well as mysticism. By posing several fundamental questions, he explains how in Islamic ethics "right and wrong" can be determined by referencing scriptural sources. In elaborating on the role of reason as well as the relationship between ethical principles, values and legal norms, the author argues that the tension and latent conflict between rules and values constitutes one of the greatest challenges to contemporary Muslim conscience.

Chapter two provides an introduction to the existing infrastructure and capacity building in Islamic bioethics. Alireza Bagheri describes how juridical supports in Islamic bioethics help to deal with newly-emerging ethical dilemmas in biomedical sciences and technologies. The chapter presents initiatives by relevant authorities in Islamic countries that have been undertaken to codify bioethical norms, guidelines or recommendations.

Chapter three presents five commentaries from Muslim, Christian and Jewish bioethicists responding to the question: what does Islamic bioethics offer to global bioethics? As an introduction to the topic, Alireza Bagheri outlines some characteristics of Islamic bioethics and the areas to which

Islamic bioethics contributes. He also provides examples where Islamic bioethics can also learn from other bioethics value systems. In his commentary Alastair Campbell elaborates first on the relationship between religion and ethics and then the similarities and differences between Islamic and Christian approaches to bioethics. He begins the exploration of the global significance of Islamic bioethics.

Carol Taylor explains the critical importance, for both Roman Catholics and Muslims, of the questions: how authoritative are moral teachings; and who is regarded as their proper interpreter. She argues that because neither the Christian Scriptures nor the Qur'an directly address many of the questions raised by today's scientific and technological advances, the question of interpretation is central. James Rusthoven reflects on the comparable struggles faced by Christian and Islamic scholars in dealing with bioethical dilemmas. He proposes that at the heart of intra-faith differences in both faith traditions is the interpretation of written Word, coloured by the historical and cultural contexts within which live people of faith. He suggests that through careful reflection and the development of solutions grounded in the Islamic faith, Muslims can make formative contributions to bioethics globally. In his commentary, Jonathan Crane, a Jewish bioethicist, contends that the global significance of Islamic bioethics is in how Islamic bioethicists continue to think deeply about the ongoing procedural connections between reason and revelation, and between ethics and law, while at the same time addressing the pressing issues of lived life. He concludes that the global need for thoughtful and responsive Islamic bioethical discourse is only increasing. Abdallah Daar asserts that the greatest challenges facing humankind today are the over-consumption of resources, degradation of the environment, threats to biodiversity, and climate change. He maintains that it is vital to seriously take up our stewardship responsibilities without delay. He further argues that the challenge of our time is to rise above and beyond narrow, parochial, tribal, obscurantist understandings and interpretations of Islam and to truly embrace the universalism already deeply rooted in Islam.

In chapter four, Ingrid Mattson elaborates on sexuality and gender identity in the Islamic context and how various Islamic discourses assert and challenge normative claims about gender and sexuality. By examining the key problematic assumptions, dominant paradigms and under-developed principles typically invoked, the author contends that the most salient feature in such discussions is the domination of the legal tradition by men. She further asserts that there is increasing evidence that significant numbers of Muslim women have participated in many fields of religious scholarship throughout Islamic history; however women authorities have been hard to find among traditional legal scholars, much less among those who have held judicial power.

Chapter five by Mohammad Albar and Hassan Chamsi-Pasha provide a clear illustration of a medical encounter in the Islamic context. They describe how a physician–patient relationship should be established and the responsibilities of physicians in Islamic society. This chapter supplies non-Muslim healthcare providers with comprehensive information for treating Muslim patients, especially women, in a multicultural society.

Abul Fadl Mohsin Ebrahim explains in chapter six how Muslim scholars have always been concerned about the determination of the end of human life as well as the consequences that follow the pronouncement of human death. He sets out the insights of Muslim scholars on the moment of death, as well as the opinions of some prominent Muslim jurists who are either for or against the utilization of human organs from brainstem-dead patients.

Chapter seven by Hakan Ertin and Ilhan Ilkilic specifies unforeseen applications of stem cell research which have posed unexpected ethical challenges to traditional views of humans and their role in the natural and divine order. The authors explain how the cultural values and religious convictions of all stakeholders involved play a decisive role in formulating ethical positions about stem cell research. They further describe the theological and philosophical criteria applied in this debate, and discuss some ethical positions formulated in the Islamic world regarding embryonic stem cell research.

Azizan Baharuddin and Mohd Noor Musa present Islamic perspectives on environmental ethics in chapter eight. They argue that according to Islam, nature has its own natural order that is regarded as the manifestation of the acts of Allah. Every element has been set to have its own functions; is also dependent on other elements; and is likewise depended upon by other elements. The authors argue that any disturbance of the natural order will cause harm to at least one component and also detrimentally affect all other elements.

Animal rights in Islam is the topic of chapter nine by Bagheri Larijani, Nazafarin Ghasemzadeh, and Mansoureh Madani. By emphasizing the sanctity of animal life and the inherent rights of animals in Islamic teachings, the chapter proposes ethical recommendations regarding the proper treatment of animals, as well as laboratory animals in biomedical research.

Mehrunisha Suleman examines biomedical research ethics in the Islamic context in chapter ten. The author describes key considerations derived from an empirical study that assesses how Islam and its normative sources influence ethical decision-making in the context of biomedical research. The chapter also provides an interesting examination of the under-studied area of women's participation in research in Islamic society.

The book concludes with an exploration by Khalid Alali, Gamal Serour and Alireza Bagheri in chapter eleven of significantly different responses to bioethical dilemmas and challenges in Islamic countries, with different levels of attention from the public, governments as well as media to various topics. The authors examine several challenges in Islamic bioethics, including: the relationship between ethics, law, and *fatwa*; the approach to principlism in Islamic bioethics; human rights in Islamic bioethics; and the lack of public awareness and participation in Islamic bioethics discourses.

Finally, we would like to thank our colleagues for their scholarly contributions to this book. Our special thanks to the anonymous reviewers; their constructive comments helped to improve the quality of the discussion in each chapter. We would also like to thank Joy Quek, the senior editor at World Scientific Publishing Co. (Singapore)

*Alireza Bagheri (Tehran, Iran)*
*Khalid Alali (Doha, Qatar)*

# References

Brockopp, J. E. 2008. Islam and Bioethics: Beyond Abortion and Euthanasia. *Journal of Religious Ethics*, 36(1), 3–12.

Campbell, A. 1999. Global Bioethics: Dream or Nightmare? *Bioethics*, 13(3/4), 183–90.

Chattopadhyay, S. and De Vries, R. 2011. Respect for Cultural Diversity in Bioethics is an Ethical Imperative. *Medicine, Health Care and Philosophy*, 16(4), 639–45.

Moazam, F. 2011. *Sharia* Law and Organ Transplantation: Through the Lens of Muslim Jurists. *Asian Bioethics Review*, 3(4), 316–32.

Murphy T. F. 2012. In Defense of Irreligious Bioethics. *American Journal of Bioethics*, 12(12), 3–10.

Sachedina, A. 2012. Defining the Pedagogical Parameters of Islamic Bioethics. *Iranian Journal of Medical Ethics*, 1(1), 34–42.

Shabana, A. 2013. Religious and Cultural Legitimacy of Bioethics: Lessons from Islamic bioethics. Medicine, *Health Care and Philosophy*, 16(4), 671–7.

Ten Have, H. and Gordijn, B. 2014. *Handbook of Global Bioethics: Introduction*. New York: Springer.

# CHAPTER ONE

# Islamic Ethics: Sources, Methodology and Application

## Tariq Ramadan

### Abstract

When discussing "Islamic ethics" it is imperative to begin by defining and describing both the terminology and the sources of ethics (*al-akhlāq*). The structure of the ethical notions in the Islamic context needs to be understood from within as well as through the evolution of what is commonly called "the Islamic sciences." This definition and identification is critical especially when our focus is on applied ethics. In Islam, ethics should be studied in relation to law and jurisprudence (*fiqh*), philosophy–theology (*kalām, falsafah*) as well as mysticism (*tasawwuf*). Drawing only on Islamic jurisprudence (*fiqh*), for example, when addressing a complex bioethical issue, may direct the analysis away from important foundational ethical discussions and fail to include Islamic philosophical and spiritual, as well as cultural, considerations.

This chapter reviews the sources of Islamic ethics as well as the methodologies used in the development of the field. Concurrently, it also examines the relationship between ethics and jurisprudence in dealing with bioethical issues.

## Introduction

The primary concern of ethics is to determine what is "good" and what is "bad." From this modest starting point, specialists in the discipline have developed a multi-faceted approach to the process of distinguishing "right" from "wrong." Systems have been established to define what can be considered as "licit" and "illicit," and will be discussed below.

*Terminology*: The discussion of ethics is broad-based, and may well lead to confusion, even among specialists, who prioritize differently the order of importance of philosophical inquiry versus legal application. Add to this, the critical debate over the sources and the origins of ethics, and of the necessary distinction that must be drawn between ethics and morals. While some believe that the only distinction is a strictly linguistic one ("ethics" being to Greek what "morals" are to Latin), philosophers and thinkers have pointed to differences of both order and nature between the two notions. Opposing views on origins (God or man); sources (revelation or reason); function (control or orientation of knowledge); and ends or "higher objectives" (divine, humanistic, utilitarian, etc.) have always been sharply demarcated. These opposing views have left their imprint on the western intellectual tradition. Positions have remained adversarial, polarized, and often irreconcilable to this day. On the one hand, there are philosophical opinions expressed by philosophers such as Paul Ricoeur and Max Weber and reaching as far back as Emmanuel Kant, Baruch Spinoza, and René Descartes. On the other hand, there are the monotheistic religions and the Greek classical tradition rediscovered by the Renaissance.

The sharp delineation of opposing views is also one of the chief hallmarks of the Islamic tradition, which subsumes a multiplicity of positions, some of which are exclusivist and even exclusionist. To grasp the nature of contemporary controversies in the Muslim world, it is essential to return to the sources, to immerse ourselves in the history of Islamic civilization. Only in this way can one understand from within the notion of "Islamic ethics" and more specifically the depth and breadth of the debates that have marked the history of Islamic thought.

There are many trends within the Islamic tradition which consider the relationship between the scriptural sources and reason. The philosophers, following in the footsteps of the Hellenic tradition, were privileging reason and the Texts were simply confirming what independent human faculty had uncovered. *Al-mu'tazila,* known as the rationalists within philosophy–theology, shared the opinion while relying more on the very scriptures to prove their points. The *Asharites* took an opposing view and refused to allow for reasoning, arguing that only the independent power determines what is right or wrong. That is, only God, hence the Qur'an, can decide and determine the ethical behaviors or acts. Al-Matūrīdī tried to find a way in between by reconciling reason and scriptures. However, the debates were at times harsh and some scholars did not hesitate to consider some of their opponents as being outside of the Islamic faith.

The very notion of ethics must be held up to close scrutiny; no exact equivalent exists in the Arabic language. Islamic legal scholars, thinkers and mystics who have grappled with the subject have by no means always agreed (not unlike in the western tradition). The two Arabic terms that best embody the notion of ethics — *akhlāq* and *adab* — share an overlapping sense of "proper conduct," of positive action and virtue. In the classical tradition, a "science of virtues" (*'ilm al-akhlāq*) quickly arose, within which legal scholars, philosophers and mystics turned their attention to matters of proper conduct, personal character, and to qualities such as self-mastery, justice and temperance, honesty, uprightness, and courage. Numerous treatises drawing on this particular definition were written in each of these fields. The notion of *adab,* which harkens back to the idea of letters and literature, quickly became associated with professional ethics and conduct. In the 11th century treatise entitled *Medical Ethics* or conduct of physicians (*Adab al-ṭabīb*), the physician Isḥāq al-Ruhāwī explores the principles that should guide the behavior of physicians (As-Saāmarraā'ī and Ar-Rahāwī, 1992). Another term, *akhlāqiyyāt,* which shares the same root as *akhlāq,* was used with increasing frequency to define the ethics of a profession or a given field of knowledge, as a replacement for *adab.*

The use of multiple terminologies, which often tells much about the extent and nature of internal discussions, leads rapidly to fundamental debates over sources as well as the formulation and status of ethics from an Islamic perspective. How, at the core of Islam, are "good" and "bad," "right" and "wrong," to be determined, and by whom? Questions include: whether reference must be made to the scriptural sources (the Qur'an and the Prophetic traditions) as a matter of priority; what is the role of reason;

what is the nature of the relationship between ethical principles and values (*akhlāq*) and legal norms (*aḥkām*); what are the connections with other religious and philosophical systems and traditions. These questions have percolated through the widely diverse circles of Muslim thought down through history, complete with — once more — a multiplicity of often-contradictory responses whether among thinkers or scholars of different Islamic sciences (law, philosophy, Sufism).

*Sources*: Ethical references are numerous in the Qur'an. Taken as a whole, the Qur'anic revelation lays down a conception of the human being: of values and ultimate goals whose core essence [deepest foundations] are of a moral order. By recognizing God and his uniqueness (*tawḥīd*), believers are called upon to choose their pathway in life by following the call to perform good deeds; to transform themselves through reform and purification; and to reject imprisonment by one's ego by possessions and by dependencies of every kind. Numerous Qur'anic verses give voice to this reality that every human being must make a choice: "By the Soul, and the proportion and order given to it. And its enlightenment as to its wrong and its right. Truly, he succeeds that purifies it. And he fails that corrupts it" (111: 7–10). Therefore, it is that one finds within itself two impulses, one toward good and the other toward evil (for thus was it created); it must then, in good conscience and in faith, choose either good or evil. That which sets the "believer" apart is a function of "good deeds," with revelation defining the faithful as "those who believe and work righteous deeds." (29: 7). It is the choice of good, on the moral level, that sets the believers apart, that allows them to accede to God's love, to paradise and to success (*falāḥ*) in this world and in the afterlife.

It is not surprising that the example to be followed by all Muslims is that of the Prophet of Islam, as set forth in the Qur'an: "We have indeed in the Apostle of God a beautiful pattern (of conduct) for any one whose hope is in God and the Final Day and who engages much in the praise of God" (33: 21). Precisely what sets the last of the Messengers, the Prophet of Islam, according to the Islamic tradition, is his moral stature, as manifested both before and during his mission. As the Qur'an reads; "And thou stands on an exalted standard of character" (68:4). The Qur'an is a message whose core and essence is the call to Mankind to recognize the existence of the Unique and to draw closer to Him by transforming oneself and one's behavior, by choosing what is right; by doing good deeds and by placing oneself at the service of justice (*'adl*). The visible expression and the social consequences of faith flow from following the example of the Prophet and "enjoining what is right (*ma'rūf*) and forbidding what is wrong (*munkar*)." When, seeking to learn more about the Prophet's character and personality, Sa'īd ibn Hishām asked the Prophet's wife, Aisha, who replied: "his character (his morality) was the Qur'an."[2] She meant that his entire being, as well as his conduct, was the manifestation of the moral teachings of Islam in every aspect of his life. By his ethical and moral carriage, he personified the message of the Qur'an.

The profoundly moral content of the Qur'an and the eminently ethical nature of the Prophet's exemplary life provide the central elements for understanding the Islamic message. Everything that is said about faith is connected with the reform and amelioration of the human being, specifically human behavior toward himself and toward nature, including animals and the planet. For the Qur'an, in emphasizing the intrinsic dignity of human beings, declares: "Now, indeed, we have conferred dignity on the children of Adam" (17: 70). Elsewhere, the quality of faith is described: "The most honored of you in the sight of God is (he who is) the most righteous."[3]

The Prophet himself was the living embodiment of the meaning of piety (*al-bir*), equating it with good conduct.[4] In a *hadith* the Prophet says: "The most perfect man in his faith, among the believers, is the one whose behavior is the most excellent (*ahsanaku-makhlâqan*)."[5] Full and consummate belief then depends upon reform of the self and of personal conduct.[6]

The close connection between faith and ethical teachings can be found at the heart of the message of Islam and has visible influences on the application of the Islamic sciences. When the Prophet explains the meaning and the essence of his mission, he states: "I have been sent to perfect [complete, bring to fruition] the most noble (*makārim*) of characters [virtues] (*al-akhlāq*)."[7] This *hadith* emphasizes that ethics is essential to values and conduct. The Prophet first affirms that the goal of his mission is to complete the teachings of his predecessors. It follows that certain values or virtues that guide humans in their conduct were already present in the religions, the spiritual traditions and the philosophies that preceded

Islam. Islam does not bring to humanity a new corpus of ethical values that replaces all that had gone before. Furthermore, the *ḥadīth* quoted above indicates that the very essence of the prophetic mission is ethical, that its intent is to teach humans higher values, and to help them to reform their conduct. It follows that the connection with God must be sought first and foremost in self-education, and that all the prescriptions (cultural practices, obligations, prohibitions) have no other aim than to reform human beings through adherence to these very values.[8] Finally, in the prophetic tradition there are two notions intimately related to the conception of Man: he is by nature "imbued with dignity (*karāmah*);" and this dignity increases through the "reverential love of God" that can only be attained through "proper conduct (*akhlāq*)." In a single, succinct formulation, the Prophet synthesized the ideal of faith, which is nothing less than the quest to attain, through personal conduct, the loftiest and most noble virtues.

## The Structure of Ethical Notions

In Islamic ethics, the prophetic tradition is of highest importance, for it indicates how the Qur'an should be read and understood. We find innumerable virtues and ethical values formulated in the Qur'an and addressed in a like number of prophetic traditions, which are directly linked to the belief in One God (*tawḥīd*). This belief extends to the fundamentals of the credo, to the regulations related to practice, and even to obligations and prohibitions. Employing a semantic analysis and a historical perspective while situating his analysis within the parameters of the Islamic system, Toshihiko Izutsu (2000) puts forward a structure of the ethical notions found in Islam. He draws on what he terms the "great moral dichotomy" that distinguishes the belief in One God (*tawḥīd*) from all other value systems (religious or profane). Beginning with *tawḥīd*, Islam presents a structure, and a corpus of values. It first distinguishes between faith (*imān*) and the negation of the Divine (*kufr*). Then it lends substance and meaning to the notions of good and bad, of the positive (*sālih*) and corruption (*fasād*), of justice (*'adl*) and injustice (*ẓulm*), of perversion (*fisq*) and purification (*tazkiyah*), and in a broader sense, that which is recognized as "good (*ma'rûf*)" from what is defined as rejected or bad in the sense of "wrong (*munkar*)."[9]

Izutsu's approach is an interesting one, but his self-enclosed, binary structure does not sufficiently recognize, or more properly, does not attach sufficient importance to Islam's recognition of universal moral values that subsumes the "great moral dichotomy" and can be located in the primordial nature of human beings themselves. Sheikh Muhammad Draz, in *The Moral World of the Qur'an*, develops a different approach, fully situated within the Islamic value system. While he examines the sources of morality, and offers a critique of the French and German philosophers Henri Bergson and Emmanuel Kant, he awards highest prominence to the idea of obligation, upon which, he argues, all moral doctrines are founded (Draz 2008, 4–16). Sheikh Draz develops a theory of the conception of Man by combining and organizing the foundational notions of Islam and returning to the scriptural sources. He argues that, there can be no ethics without the faculty of reason necessary to not only grasp the "obligation (*farīḍah*)," but also the "responsibility (*mas'ūliyyah*)." Autonomous reason, in the Kantian sense, is insufficient; instead, only a superior form of "reason" that is not "transcendental" but "Transcendent" (God) can provide coherence to the entire edifice of morality (Draz 2008, 14). The light of humanity thus encounters the Light of the Divine — as found in the Qur'anic verse, "Light upon light" (24: 35), through which Man can develop a moral doctrine founded upon certain, immutable and universal values. As we see, unlike Izutsu, Draz's position is antecedent to the "moral dichotomy" that would distinguish between human beings. He expounds instead a description of Man while detailing the common — universal — underpinnings that make it possible to explain the Islamic doctrine. This doctrine begins with initial responsibility and is articulated around freedom, sanction, intention and effort as applied to every sphere of applied ethics at the individual, family, social, state, and religious levels (Draz 2008, 100, 196). Ethical values can thus claim two sources. The first is Man, who in his primordial nature, his *fiṭrah* (which is neither fundamentally good nor fundamentally bad) relies upon his reason, finding in it "the brotherhood of man;"[10] and the second, beyond it, by way of revelation, common ethical and universal values laid down by both human and transcendent Divinity.

These two contemporary readings of the Qur'an command attention in several ways — as both aspire to present either a theory of Islamic ethics drawing on structures inherent in Islam (and of the Arabic language) or a theory based on an understanding of universal ethics. Both provide an excellent introduction to the way in which, over the centuries, Muslim scholars and thinkers have approached the question of ethics. Three factors have played a significant role in the reading and interpretation of the scriptural sources. First, the area of specialization of the scholars and thinkers who delved into the subject; their values; and finally the significance of prescriptions and their ultimate goals directly influenced several of the "Islamic sciences" (primarily law, mysticism, and philosophy). Thus, the organization of the value structure is heavily influenced by the legal, metaphysical or spiritual approach to the subject. Secondly, the historical circumstances and internal debates within Muslim communities should not be overlooked. Relationships between political power, religious institutions, as well as internal conflicts between schools of thought and jurisprudence all had an impact on the way moral values were understood, organized and applied. Lastly, Islam's relationship with other religious, spiritual or philosophical traditions cannot be minimized. These relationships were to determine the moral discourse against which thinkers would position themselves or seek connections with other referential universes. It should be noted that moral theories and ethical concepts do not spring from a void. They are directly connected — above and beyond the founding texts — to the thinkers who conceived them; to the internal dynamics of their systems of reference as well as to their relationships with other religions and philosophies.

## Typology of Sciences

Islamic ethics has been influenced by internal and external historical factors in its formulation and constitution, and its relation to other fields of knowledge. By virtue of its direct connection with the interpretation of the founding scriptural sources, Islamic ethics is integrated naturally from three distinct fields: that of law and jurisprudence (*fiqh*); philosophy and theology; and mysticism (*taṣawwuf*). The three fields, together, separately or in opposition to one another, produced a broad range of moral theories as well as the diverse ethical systems that lie at the heart of the Muslim tradition.

In his *Ethical Theories in Islam*, Majid Fakhry (1994) lays out a typology that follows, in its broad outline, that put forward by George F. Hourani (1985) in his *Reason and Tradition in Islamic Ethics*. Fakhry defines ethics as "scriptural morality," which directly presents in the texts, and precedes the construction of any conceptual structure. However, three other fields of research later emerged. The first Hourani defines as "theological theory" which Islamic theologians[11] discussed as the role of reason within Islam. The second was "philosophical theory" developed by philosophers influenced by the Hellenic tradition. Finally, the third was "religious theory" that was presented as the work and reflection of scholars reading the texts. These scholars were, directly or indirectly, influenced by Greek or Christian scholars.[12]

Such a typology is, however, problematic for at least three reasons. First, categories of this kind, which are often comprehensible and justifiable, encounter difficulties when they come up against the transversal debates that touch not only upon questions of religion, but also upon those of theology and philosophy. Historically, theories and intellectual exchange were never compartmentalized and a classification system of this kind is not always consistent with the historical era in which the scholars lived, their religious concerns, and the political world they inhabited. Secondly, the specific subjects and the obstacles upon which scholars based their agreements and disagreements are not always clearly stated. Finally, as Hourani and Fakhry themselves recognize, they have omitted the mystical tradition, while it was precisely this tradition that most strongly contributed to the articulation of the ethical values and proper conduct that lie at the heart of the Muslim tradition.

The typology put forward here is slightly different. While not denying the need to categorize and classify or to draw up a coherent typology of ethical theories in Islam, the aim instead is to simplify and simultaneously clarify the question. The point of common ground from which views diverge, as always, must be the unanimously recognized texts that provide the subject matter of all the Islamic sciences. Secondly, the different modes of appreciation and interpretation of the texts, within the limited purview of those sciences that touch upon ethics, must be established. Only then will it be possible to grasp the nature of the conflicting points of view inherent in each, along with the different methodologies put forward within each science: law, theology–philosophy and mysticism. Particularly revealing is the nature of the doubts often expressed with regard to the scriptural sources about which consensus exists. The highly specific nature of these doubts, and the methodologies put forward to answer them according to the sciences in question, is striking. It should come as no surprise that Islamic jurists were interested in understanding the texts and in deriving ethical values and rules of conduct from them. Their approach — once the authenticity of the sources had been recognized — was one of explanation and description. Differences of opinion between jurists and schools of law and jurisprudence were primarily over the status of the texts and methodologies used to understand them (in their literal meaning, with the interpretative scope they offer, or in their silence) and to derive rules from them. The doubts expressed by the partisans of theologians, philosophers, and by Muslim philosophers influenced by the Greeks, inspired efforts to determine the origin and the sources of moral values from the scriptural sources. In constructing an ethical system, scholars considered what is the portion of the divine, and what is that of the human being. The goal, for them, was not simply to understand the texts, but to determine the extent of human autonomy with regard both to the scriptural sources and in constructing a value system.

## Law and Jurisprudence (*Fiqh*) and the Sources

As this chapter is an introduction to Islamic ethics in the light of bioethics, it is the field of jurisprudence that is the most related to bioethics (even though the two others contribute significantly in philosophical and spiritual terms). A close reading of the Qur'an and the Prophetic traditions (*sunna*), reveals a substantial number of ethical values presented in the Qur'anic verses, through the stories related and the subjects explored. They are naturally, though not exclusively, connected with certain legal prescriptions concerning worship ('*ibādāt*) or social affairs (*mu'āmalāt*), and have a broader impact. The earliest jurists, from all the schools of jurisprudence, *Sunnī* and *Shī'a*, evoked these values as they sought to understand the rules (*ahkām*), their application (*taḍbīq*), and/or their ultimate goals (*maqāsid*). It seemed clear to them that the understanding of rules and regulations, and their meaning, was linked — explicitly or not — to a moral outlook and framework. The first collection of *aḥādīth*, (plural *hadith*) which at the same time was a book of *fiqh*, provides a fascinating example. In fact, the book of *al-Muwaṭṭa* of Imām Mālik (d. 795), is not limited to a compilation of Prophetic traditions. It includes the opinions of the companions and the guarantors of knowledge (*ahl al-'ilm*) of the city of Medina and describes the manners and customs of the town (*Sunna*) and the views of imam Mālik himself on certain questions. This first compendium of law and jurisprudence written by Imam al-Shāfi'ī (which precedes the synthesis of the methodology of law and its objectives) approaches questions from a thoroughly practical angle (Dutton 1999). According to this book which is considered as the exclusive content of the *sunna*, the ethics of conduct is what is naturally recognized (*ma'rūf*) by the inhabitants of Medina. Proper conduct and the meaning of prescriptions are to be interpreted in the light of life as it is lived, according to the goals of activity, while ethical considerations are integrated into a thought process that goes beyond the transcription of narrated rules (*aḥādīth*). Al-Shāfi'ī's chapter on ethics deals specifically with proper conduct and noble character but his overall approach brings together, in a natural way, rules and regulations (*aḥkām*), the life-style of the people of Medina (as a source) and the ultimate ethical goals that lend meaning to the message as a whole. The first objective is to concentrate on the activity — taken in concrete terms — upon which moral values confer meaning; which rules and regulations lend structure; and towards what objectives it guides. *Fiqh*, since its inception and in the manner in which it deals with the sources (and primarily the *Sunna*), appears to enjoy an ethical and juridical function, one that links rules to norms, and which stands, *de facto*, as the first expression of applied Islamic ethics.

## Legal Tools and Ethics

At the very heart of the process of drafting Islamic law, it is important to identify general principles based on practical rationality and attention to the meanings and ethical objectives of the law. Certainly, legal rulings enjoyed predominance, and their moral implications, were neither entirely absent nor neglected. Seen in this light, the five categories of rules governing the legal and ethical value of human activity as a whole (*aḥkām at-taklīfiyya*) may be taken as strictures of an ethico-legal nature and consist of the permitted (*mubāḥ*); the obligatory (*wājib*); the preferable (*mustaḥab*); the reprehensible (*makrūh*); and the forbidden (*ḥarām*). In fact, legal scholars never abandoned their interest in the question of what constitutes the good, the positive, the just, the acceptable, etc. Scholars also considered the objectives of action as seen through the prism of ethical values. Although the extraction of rules remained a priority, partly because of scholarly specialization, the question of ethics remained central to the legal categorization of human actions. The same reference to values can also be observed in the work of deducing, understanding and applying rules in a given era, geographical or cultural context. The search for the primary reason for a particular rule (*'illa*), which can be explicit, suggested or absent, obliged scholars to consider in their deliberations the intentions and moral objectives associated with a rule (*ḥukm*), or the justification for their legal opinions (*fatwā*).

Concentration on a legalistic and formalized expression of a rule to the exclusion of all else tended to skew the necessary balance between formulation and full consideration of its ethical significance. However, as the source of the rule extraction process (*istinbāṭ*), the law cannot exist without ethics, nor the rule without moral value. The tension and latent conflict between rules and values constitutes one of the greatest challenges to contemporary Muslim conscience. Furthermore, the practice of autonomous ethical and legal reasoning (*ijtihād*), obliges legal scholars to refer constantly to the higher moral values and the rationality of the Qur'anic message especially when the texts are mute or open to interpretation, or when applying rules to a specific context (such as bioethics). Therefore, *ijtihād* cannot be undertaken in a coherent manner without full awareness of the ultimate goals of the law and of the moral structure that underlies it.

## Fiqh and Sharī'a

Alongside the evolution in thought that restricted the meaning of certain key notions, such as *Sunna* to *aḥādīth* in their legal dimensions — or *fiqh* — to law and ethics — the very notion of *Shari'a* experienced a contraction and a narrowed interpretation. Beginning with the exercise of *fiqh* and its focus on laws and rules, *Shari'a* came to be defined first, as "Islamic law" and second as the founding corpus of immutable laws (*thābit*); or as the "incontrovertible law of God." As a result, the contraction of *Shari'a* had a far greater impact than the previous two definitions, as discussed. Some Islamic scholars have called this reductionism into question. They have suggested that *Sharî'a* needs a more holistic understanding and definition.

Al-Rāghib al-Isfahānī (d. 1108), the theologian–philosopher and Qur'anic commentator, authored the book with the evocative title *The Path Towards Shari'a's Virtues (al-Dharī'ailā Makārim al-Shari'a)*. This work is a major contribution to the understanding of *Shari'a* and the role of the diverse sciences that brought it into being (Al-Isfahānī 1987). His thesis can be better understood by first analyzing what he posits as the ultimate goal of creation and, through it, interpreting the teachings of *Shari'a*. That goal, he argues, is the establishment of a civilization on earth that respects the Qur'anic message and brings about the Vicegerency (*khilāfa*) of mankind. Vicegerency in turn is based on recognition of the presence of God (*tawḥīd*) and the efforts of mankind to apply divine prescriptions and to respect values and rules, both individually and collectively, in every facet of life. The idea of *khilāfa* is not merely political, but closely related to the life of mankind through the prism of faith in God. It brings mankind closer to God through the attainment of two virtues which are central principles: justice and love.[13] Al-Rāghib al-Isfahānī's approach to *Shari'a* understood, as the realization of the ultimate goal of creation, is both broad and open: human beings are summoned to draw closer to the Divine out of respect for revelation, for reason and for the heart.

Upon understanding the ultimate goal, it becomes easier to understand the noble virtues of the *Shari'a* to which the title refers. The core essence for strict religious observance is the imperative respect for the prescribed rules. Only upon fulfillment of this condition can man develop the other essential component of complete Vicegerency. Only through spiritual exercise, moral purification, and reform (*islāḥ*) of one's character and conduct, may man accede to religious nobility. Inductively, law, and ethics are thus reconciled; Vicegerency is possible only through the marriage of both norm and virtue.

The *Mālikī* and *Ash'arī* legal scholar AbūIsḥāqIq al-Shātibī (d. 1388) advanced a new approach to the understanding of law and jurisprudence (*fiqh*) and its fundamentals (*uṣūl al-fiqh*) by concentrating on the objectives of *Sharī'a*. Like al-Isfahānī before him, al-Shātibī set forth a typology of the ultimate goals of *Sharī'a* (*maqāsid al-Sharī'a*). By concentrating on looking beyond the literal meaning of a given rule he sought the aims of the Islamic message (by type and by order of priority) that link all the sciences, and, above all, law and ethics. Al-Shātibī's approach was to stimulate a renewed sense of dynamism among scholars and Muslims of the day. Scholars from all schools of jurisprudence were both attentive to and worried by the hyper-development of the law and its predominance over all the other sciences, particularly with regard to the study of ethical values, spirituality, and proper conduct. More than a few of them questioned the modalities of reading the scriptural sources, while others sought to bring the ultimate goals of the message to the fore. The central issue in both pursuits was this: in order to achieve the plenitude of the message, the use of reason based upon revelation and the Prophetic tradition (*Sunna*) is required to understand the law.

## Applied Ethics

Islam, like all other religions, grappled with the emergent scientific and technological issues as well as the progress and evolution of sciences. Islamic jurists have essentially, taken this task upon themselves. Over time, they have promulgated legal rulings and judicial opinions (*fatāwā*) on objects, actions, and situations that cannot be resolved by reference to the Qur'an or the *Sunna*. This method of judicial exercise has existed since the very origins of Islam, and is known as *ijtihād*: when legal scholars working in the field of social affairs (*mu'āmalāt*) produce an informed opinion (*fatwa*) on a given subject where the texts are either open to interpretation or silent. Three important points must be made: firstly, *ijtihād* is an exercise in legal reasoning, individual or collective, carried out in the spirit of the texts and the overreaching ultimate ethical goals of the message. Secondly, it is imperative that those responsible for legal rulings fully master the fields of knowledge (medicine, economy, the environment, etc.) in which they will be setting down guidelines and limits. Thirdly, the legal rulings produced are by definition neither exhaustive nor restrictive. Individuals in their private lives and scientists, in the practice of their professions, must choose according to the dictates of personal conscience. Nevertheless, *ijtihād* requires more than only reacting to the state of affairs in specific scientific fields but also anticipating ethical issues. Considering ethical values as well as the higher objectives (*maqāsid*), it means having to go beyond the detailed response on a specific issue. The overall development in the scientific field in question should also be considered in a prospective way. Ethical questioning changes the nature of legal reasoning (*ijtihād fiqhī*) by requiring a holistic approach to determining the ends of the scientific knowledge itself, and not only attending to the structural protective function of law.

The concentration of ethical inquiry and elucidation in the hands of legal scholars can be explained by the development of Islamic sciences and their accompanying hierarchical structure, as described above. Nonetheless, it is clear that general ethical reflection, when it becomes a strictly legalistic examination whose only aim is to determine the licit (*halāl*) and the illicit (*harām*), will be reduced to an exercise in jurisprudence that attends to novelty in detail but is unable to grasp the breadth and complexity of new situations created by scientific progress. A legalistic examination, therefore, neglects not only the paradigms that govern new ways of understanding, but also the theory of knowledge that generates meaning and the ethical questions generated by social, scientific, and intellectual development. Worse yet, these Islamic scholars more often lack a basic grasp and informed overview of the scientific elements and of the theoretical and practical information on the topics under discussion. Their overview (in both conceptual and temporal terms) of the subject is often deficient and uninformed by a holistic vision. Consequently, their rulings are based on a partial understanding of the specifics or of a given set of circumstances. In contrast, *ijtihād*, as practiced by judicial councils (*al-majālis al-fiqhiyyah*), strives to remain current with the evolution of knowledge and practice. It establishes limits derived from experience (the nature of all jurisprudence), but possesses neither the competence nor the time for serious examination of the structure inherent in the means and objectives of science and technology themselves. It should be noted that with a handful of rare exceptions, scientists are absent from these legal and ethical deliberations, while thinkers and philosophers are all but excluded. However, compartmentalization has trapped ethics within legality, while legality has become subservient to the jurisprudence of practical detail and is cut off from the broad view of theory. The positive aspect is that legal opinions so expressed have no constraining force; individuals and societies must follow the dictates of their conscience. More problematic, however, is what could be termed a double relegation of ethical considerations in the minds of Muslims. Not only does the legal (or non-legal) character of a decision take precedence in directing or orienting action but, in addition, the non-constraining nature of any given ruling relieves the individual of the responsibility of ethical reflection. Over-regulation by law, which should lend weight to applied ethics, ends up paradoxically reducing ethics to a secondary matter, given that law and jurisprudence are unable to express a single, definitive or constraining opinion. Thus the process of juridical decision-making, while dynamic and flexible in matters of detail, ultimately works against engendering respect for the higher ethical principles that should bind mankind's conscience and spirituality. The phenomenon can be observed in virtually all fields of knowledge, but for this chapter we will restrict ourselves to the revealing case of medicine. Medicine is the field in which Muslim scholars have made the greatest progress, both in juridical–ethical investigation and working methods. Progress, in terms of both knowledge and of medical technology, has been so great and so rapid that it has become imperative to devise new ways of anticipating problems formulating legal rulings governing the licit or illicit character of any particular procedure or practice. Islamic jurists have conceded the limits of their medical knowledge while, at the same time, more and more Muslim physicians have found themselves thrust into situations that either raised questions of conscience or conflicted directly with their professional principles. While the latter seek answers consistent with the precepts of Islam, the former require the counsel of specialized practitioners to provide the information needed to formulate applicable legal rulings. Joint consultative councils, in which legal scholars join forces with physicians, have been created in several countries, notably in Kuwait. Since 1981, the Islamic Organization of Medical Science (IOMS), makes it possible to obtain legal rulings that are fully informed by contemporary medical discoveries and practices. These extremely diversified and at times contradictory rulings (according to the Councils cited) touch on virtually all fields of medical knowledge: life, death, health, bioethics, and the most advanced medical technology

(Ramadan 2008). In the minutes of their working meetings, legal scholars and physicians can be observed discussing end-of-life issues. For example, brain death, euthanasia, the principles and methods of *in vitro* fertilization, cloning, abortion, organ transplants, research on bioethics, the human genome, and bioethics itself (IOMS 1981–1999). In those efforts, specific answers were provided to each of these issues. Sometimes unanimous, sometimes endorsed by a simple majority, the legal opinions demonstrate that jurists are quite capable of grappling with complex issues such as euthanasia, *in vitro* fertilization, therapeutic cloning, and abortion on a case-by-case basis. Their decisions are exhaustively argued, determined by specific circumstances, and have the merit of providing both practitioners and patients with detailed, up-to-date guidance.

Nonetheless, the field of medicine and bioethics, the most advanced in terms of applied Islamic ethics, reveals at least four difficulties symptomatic of the evolution of contemporary Muslim thought, which are pertinent to all fields of knowledge. First, due to the language barrier, the legal opinions (which are mostly in Arabic) are unfortunately little publicized and narrowly disseminated. Thus, many physicians and scientists as well as the public are unaware of the advances in Islamic thought as applied to medical ethics and bioethics. In addition, there is no specific training program for physicians in Islamic jurisprudence, and therefore understanding legal rulings can often be problematic. Furthermore, many physicians or scientists view the ethical aspects as a secondary consideration. Second, these legal rulings, which can be extremely specific and detailed, often overlook fundamental realities such as the relationship of medicine to the economy and the pharmaceutical industry; social justice; equitable access to healthcare; the use of personal data; etc. However, formulating a legal ruling on the end of life, euthanasia, organ transplantation, or cloning without taking into account the many complexities of the economic, cultural, and political power structures represents a serious and even grave deficiency. Unfortunately, legal scholars are not always ualified to evaluate the wider consequences of their specialized and specific rulings.

The third difficulty arises from the approach itself, with respect to the current holistic vision of the multi-dimensional human person. If applied ethics is viewed uniquely through the prism of the legal, the licit and the illicit, then it is not possible to examine contemporary medical science; the definitions of health and illness; the techniques utilized; and the remedies administered. Issues of death and suffering and the treatments for palliation are today considered part of the normal, and normalized, evolution of science and technology. At a seminar on bioethics[14] organized by the Centre for Islamic Legislation and Ethics (CILE), the participants, legal scholars, medical practitioners, and philosophers discussed the four guiding principles of biomedical ethics — autonomy, justice, beneficence, and non-maleficence (Beauchamp and Childress 1979) — the central question was that of life itself. In reaction to the extremely technical nature of the debate over the prevention of suffering, a Muslim scholar insisted on the primary necessity to define health and life. Fundamental reflections of this nature, however, tend to be absent from exchanges among legal scholars. For example, the philosophical grounding and the ultimate goals that confer meaning upon the human person and the medical act are rarely or not at all taken into consideration. The usual imperative is to formulate a practical answer to a concrete case. Everything else is little more than "philosophy."

To this list must be added a fourth difficulty, which is closely tied to the Islamic world's relations with the West. In most discussions about medical ethics and bioethics, participants situate themselves relative not only to a particular area of knowledge or technique, but also to the dominant western approach to bioethics. Depending on the subject under study, relations with the West play a key role in determining how questions are answered and legal rulings are formulated.

## Conclusion

Applied Islamic ethics, as developed almost exclusively by legal scholars in all scientific disciplines, suffers from these four problems: the language barrier; overlooking the relationship between medicine, economy, and social justice; dominance of the legal approach to applied ethics; as well as the Islamic world's relations with the West. The channels of communication and collaboration between legal scholars and specialized experts (i.e., physicians, economists, environmentalists) are severely limited, as are interactions with the specialists of other religious traditions or those who are atheist or agnostic. It is essential to revisit and reexamine a multiplicity of core concepts, including those of *Sharī'a*, ethics, *ratio legis* (*manāṭ*), interest (*masālih*) and objectives (*maqāsid*), as well as the idea of reform (*iṣlāḥ*) itself. In spiritual and ethical terms, it is important to consider whether the choice lies between reforming interpretations to better adapt to scientific progress and the evolution of the world, or renewing our understanding of the texts to better reform and transform the world for the better. Many scholars and thinkers use the term reform but cannot agree upon either its meaning or its implications. Some speak of adaptive reform. Most Islamic jurists (*faqih*) belong to this category since law and jurisprudence, by their nature, can adapt to changed circumstances. Others, however, conceive of an inherent exigency accompanied by a process of transformation of the world in the light of ethics and ultimate goals. Not only legal scholars should participate in the process of ethical enquiry, but also philosophers, mystics, and scientists of both genders. The road will be arduous and filled with numerous obstacles to success. Over the course of centuries entire fields of knowledge have become circumscribed and compartmentalized; incestuous relationships with power have emerged, and prerogatives (in terms of legal and ethical authority) have become institutionalized. Only a rethinking of ethics, starting with a renewed conception of man and the universe (*fiṭrah, khilāfah*) and concluding with ultimate goals, while rejecting the exclusive preeminence of law, can shake the old order and weaken the reflexes developed over centuries.

## Notes

[1] According to Qur'anic verse 22: 41.
[2] *Ḥadīth* reported by Muslim, Abū Dawūd and Aḥmad.
[3] *Atqākum* here refers to the polysemic notion of *taqwā*, meaning awareness of God, piety, and the love and reverential fear of God.
[4] *Ḥadīth* reported by Muslim.
[5] *Ḥadīth* reported by Bukhārī and Muslim.
[6] *Ḥadīth* reported by at-Tirmidhī (*ḥassan-saḥīḥ*).
[7] *Ḥadīth* reported by Mālik and Aḥmad.
[8] The source of Ibn al-Qayyim's famous formula: "All religion is ethical (proper conduct, virtues)."

[9] Each of these terms is polysemic; Izutsu exercises great care and takes considerable time to define and to situate the moral values enumerated within his proposed general structure.

[10] Here Draz refers to the notion of "human brotherhood."

[11] Majid Fakhry's definition; they are better described as belonging to two fields of knowledge, as "theologian–philosophers."

[12] In his book, Hourani speaks of "normative religious ethics" and of "secular normative ethics" and suggests a single line to demarcate the religious, the theological, and the philosophical, *op. cit.*, pp. 15–22.

[13] Al-Rāghib al-Isfahānī describes this notion in greater depth in another work on ethics: *Taḥsīl al-Nash'ataynwaTaḥsīl al-Sa'adatyan* (*Exposition of the Two Births and Acquisition of the Two Felicities*), ed. A. Najjar. Beirut : al-matba'a al-'arabiyya, 1988.

[14] Seminar on Bioethics and Universal Principles (Doha, January 5–7, 2013). Participants: Prof. Tom Beauchamp, Dr. Annelien Bredennoord, Dr. Muhammad Ali Albar, Shaykhar-Raysūnī, Shaykh 'Abd al-Sattar, AbūGhudda, Shaykh Ali al-Quaradāghī.

## References

Al-Isfahānī R. 1987. *Al-Dharī'ailā Makārim al-Sharī'a*. Abū al-Yazīd al-'Ajamī (ed.). Cairo: Dār al-kutub al-'ilmiyya. See also thesis by Yasien M. 2006. *The Path of Virtue: The Ethical Philosophy of Al-Rāghib al-Isfahānī*. Kuala Lumpur: International Institute of Islamic Thought and Civilization.

As-Sāmarrāī Kamāl and Ar-Rahāwī Isḥāq Ibn-Alī. 1992. *Kitāb adab at-tabīb* (1992 ed.).

Baghdād: Dāras-Suūnat-Thaqāfīyaal-Āmma Āfāq Arabīya".

Beauchamp, T. L. and Childress, J. F. 1979. *Principles of Biomedical Ethics*. New York: Oxford University Press. See also Beauchamp, T. L. 2011. *Standing on Principles: Collected Essays*. New York: Oxford University Press.

Draz, M. 2008. *The Moral World of the Qur'an*. London: I. Tauris.

Dutton, Y. 1999. *The Origins of Islamic Law: The Qur'an, the Muwatta' and Madinan Amal*. London: Routledge.

Fakhry, M. 1994. *Ethical Theories in Islam*. Leiden: Brill.

Hourani, G. F. 1985. *Reason and Tradition in Islamic Ethics*. Cambridge: Cambridge University Press.

Imām Mālik Ibn Anas. [Undated]. *Al-Muwaṭṭa*. Kuala Lumpur: Islamic Book Trust.

Islamic Organization for Medical Sciences (IOMS). 1981–1999. *The Islamic Vision of Some Medical Practices.* Kuwait City: IOMS.

Izutsu, T. 2000. *The Structuré of Ethical Terms in the Qur'an.* Chicago: ABC International Group Inc.

Ramadan, T. 2008. *Radical Reform* (Section Four, on case studies, medicine in particular, Chapter 11). New York: Oxford University Press.

# CHAPTER TWO

## Islamic Bioethics: Infrastructure and Capacity Building

### *Alireza Bagheri*

### Summary

A quarter of the world's population are Muslims. For many Muslims either living in Muslim countries or in non-Muslim countries, religious law is a major factor in healthcare decision-making and has traditionally provided the foundation for policy development. Recently, in Islamic countries, bioethics, as an academic discipline, has been gaining more attention in medicine, law and Islamic jurisprudence. With the increasing interest in Islamic bioethics, many Islamic countries have developed programs to build capacity to deal with bioethical issues in the Islamic context.

As a religious-based bioethics, Islamic bioethics collaborates closely with Islamic jurisprudence in ethical deliberations that guide human action, resolve ethical dilemmas, and make significant recommendations for healthcare providers, policy-makers as well as the public.

This chapter describes existing bioethics resources as well as initiatives in developing Islamic bioethics capacity in Muslim societies.

## Introduction: Religious-Based Bioethics

Islam has the second largest religious affiliation across the world which includes a quarter of the world's population. With increased migration, the

Muslim population is scattered around the world, and a large number of Muslims now live in non-Muslim countries. Thus, understanding Muslim religious law and ethics is critical for healthcare professionals when addressing healthcare needs of a Muslim patient.

The Prophet of Islam announced the perfection of morals as the aim of his appointment as the messenger of God (Abu Abdallah Muhammad 1002). In Islamic teachings, the importance of inter-human as well as human-divine relations has been emphasized. Muslims look at these teachings to shape their relationship with others and the Almighty God. For many Muslims, whether living in Muslim countries or in non-Muslim countries, the teachings of Islam have shaped their personal social life as well as their practice and attitude towards health, illness, life, and death. In healthcare decision-making, especially in issues related to the beginning of life as well as the end of life, religious law is a major determinant for Muslims. Furthermore, Islamic legal and ethical traditions form the foundation of inquiries around new emerging issues in the field of biomedicine (Shomali 2008) and cover practical aspects of clinical and research-related decision-making. Muslim ethics tries to make sense of human moral instincts, institutions, and traditions in order to provide a foundation of rules and principles that can govern a virtuous life (Sachedina 2009, 25).

Although Islamic countries are geographically diverse, they are nevertheless similar in terms of religious background. In Islamic societies, bioethical discussions and related policy-making are inspired by Islamic moral teachings and based on Islamic ethics. In Islamic jurisprudence, if there is no textual ordinance (*nass*) offering explicit guidance on the issue under consideration, decisions on the matter fall within the domain of juristic discretion (*ijtihad*). In the absence of a central authority for all schools of thought in Islam, determination of valid religious practice is left to the opinion of qualified scholars of Islamic *Shari'a* (*faqih*). In dealing with bioethical questions, it has been argued that respect for Islamic religious norms is essential for the legitimacy of bioethical standards in the Muslim context (Shabana 2013). In practice, Islamic scholars and institutions are therefore involved in bioethical discussions on issues such as abortion, artificial reproductive technologies, brain death, and organ transplantation. In summary, it can be claimed that in many Islamic societies bioethics is dominated by legal rulings (*fatwa*) of Islamic jurisprudence.

## Juridical Support to Deal with Newly-Emerging Issues

In Islamic jurisprudence, the ethical dilemmas that accompany the progress of human knowledge and technology are considered as newly-emerging issues.

The foundational source in the gradual codification of Islamic ethics is the Muslim understanding and interpretations of the Qur'an and practices of the Prophet (Shapiro *et al.* 2015). Islamic regulations are originally expressed as specific general principles and norms, which are not expounded in detail. Therefore, in dealing with bioethical issues raised by new technologies, there is often a lack of textual ordinance and explicit guidance in the primary sources of Islamic jurisprudence, the Qur'an and the *Sunna*. These issues are the matters that fall within the domain of legal discretion (*ijtihad*). To obtain an Islamic opinion (*fatwa*) for an ethical dilemma in medicine, for example, whether organ removal following brain death is permissible, these steps are followed. First, medical specialists explain the problem of brain death and the state and conditions of the patient to an Islamic jurist (*faqih*), and pose their question. Then the *faqih* utilizes authentic sources and documents that include the Qur'an and the *Sunna* as the main primary sources of Islamic *Shari'a*. When the Islamic opinion is expressed by a *faqih*, it is called a *fatwa*, which is a non-binding legal opinion. Muslim physicians then perform their medical duties according to these expressed legal opinions and recommendations. In practice, a constructive collaboration between Islamic jurists (experts of the Texts) and medical specialists (experts of the context) is very critical to resolve such complex questions. Leading juridical authorities in different centers of Islamic learning have participated in formulating religious responses to the emerging problems created by the phenomenal advancement in biotechnology and medical practice. It should be noted that in Islamic law controversy exists not only among different schools of thought such as *Shi'a* and *Sunni*, but also within each of these schools. For instance, different ruling *fatwas* on the application of assisted reproductive technologies and abortion can be seen among *Shi'a* scholars and *Sunni* scholars (Bagheri and Afshar 2011). It should be noted that, in many Islamic countries like Saudi Arabia, Iran, and Turkey, some *fatwas* as well as bioethical recommendations have become parliamentary legislations.

## Islamic Bioethics: Infrastructure and Institutions

Islamic organizations in their national, regional and international capacity have created an institutional infrastructure to address bioethical issues in the Islamic context. For instance the Organization of the Islamic Cooperation (OIC) and the Islamic Educational, Scientific and Cultural Organization (ISESCO) provide bioethical guidance which impact all Islamic Member States. These organizations have an important legitimizing effect, yet their recommendations are also subject to debate and dissent. Norm-production, therefore, depends on the cogency of argument, the clarity of precedent, and the power to make one's voice heard.

The Islamic Juridical Council of the Muslim World League in Mecca (*Majma'al-Fiqh al-Islami*) discussed many critical issues in medical ethics (Albar and Chamsi-Pasha 2015). For instance the Council has issued rulings such as: the use of alcohol, porcine material, and blood in medicine (1981); contraception (1980); *in vitro* fertilization (1982); brain death and organ transplantation (1985); post mortem examination (1987); issues related to inter-sex and trans-sex (1989); abortion with specific reference to congenital anomalies (1990).

In 1985, following early interest in bioethical issues, Islamic governments formed an advisory body called the International Islamic Juridical Council that functions under the Organization of Islamic Cooperation (OIC). One of the main tasks of the Council is to study ethical issues in biomedicine. Apart from cross-national initiatives to deal with bioethical issues, many Islamic countries have established national bioethics and medical ethics academic centers. These centers have developed bioethics educational and research programs and are in consultative relationships with relevant authorities making bioethics-related laws and regulations. For instance, in Iran, the Center for Medical Ethics and History of Medicine in Tehran Medical University has developed national ethical guidelines for clinical trials, genomic research, organ transplantation, stem cell therapy, and animal research (http://mehr.tums.ac.ir/Codes.aspx?lang=en).

In Kuwait, since 1981, the Islamic Organization for Medical Sciences has studied ethical perspectives in medicine. During its first International Conference on Islamic Medicine, members adopted the "Islamic Code of Medical Ethics" as well as the "Oath of a Muslim Physician." In this oath, which is similar to Hippocratic Oath with minor differences, physicians swear: "To be ever-conscious of my duty to Allah and His Messenger and to follow the precepts of Islam in private and in public." It continues, "O Allah grant me the strength, patience and dedication to adhere to this Oath at all times."

Since 2000, each medical school in Indonesia has established a bioethics unit and developed an ethics curriculum for medical students. As for postgraduate studies, the school of medicine at the University of Gadja Mada offers a Masters program in bioethics. Indonesia is now part of the University Bioethics and Humanities Education Network which is an international partnership in bioethics education among several Asian, European, and American universities. The Indonesian National Bioethics Committee was established in 2004, and in 2005 the National Commission of Health Research Ethics began its activity. Currently all health institutions have an Institutional Review Board (Sastrowijoto *et al.* 2014)

In Saudi Arabia, since 2009, the King Saud bin Abdulaziz University for Health Sciences offers a Masters in Bioethics. The program aims to reinforce Islamic perspectives on the ethics of medical practice. The program seeks to explore the most important ethical problems in the health fields, and to develop a vision on how to deal with those problems in the present and future. Medical ethics courses are part of medical school curriculums and in some medical schools, such as the College of Medicine at King Saud University, medical ethics is taught in two courses. One course in the first year covers topics such as patients' rights, Islamic medical ethics, and Islamic ethical principles. The second course in the third year focuses more on practical issues such as brain death, organ transplantation, and abortion.

In Turkey, the Turkish Bioethics Association established in 1994 is a leading force behind the development of bioethics at the national level. The Society for Medical Ethics and Medical Law as well as the Ethics Committee of the Turkish Medical Association are other national bodies working on bioethical issues. In 1991, bioethics committees were established following a public discussion on the issue of ethical norms in medical research. Since 1961, all medical schools have a Medical Deontology Course which was modified in 1981 to become the Medical Ethics Course. The National Bioethics Committee was established in 2000 under the UNESCO National Commission (Arda 2014).

In Yemen, the Aden Medical School has been a pioneer in medical ethics education for undergraduates since 1975. Later on, in 2003, it introduced ethics courses into the postgraduate curriculum (Hattab and Ramon 2004).

In Egypt, the International Islamic Center for Population Studies and Research in Al-Azhar University is a leading center which established the first bioethics committee in 1991 and developed the bioethics curriculum in 2000. Ain-Shams University, in collaboration with Maryland University, developed a program on bioethics committees and ethics in research specifically to build capacity in research ethics (Ragab 2015). It is worth mentioning that the rulings of the Grand Muftis of Egypt on medical and health issues, which have been collected and published, are also a significant source for medical jurisprudence and bioethics in many Islamic countries.

In Lebanon, the Salim El-Hoss Bioethics and Professionalism Program was established in 2010 in the American University of Beirut. The center is involved in bioethics education, research, and consultation in Lebanon and the region. It aims to enhance public awareness and understanding as well as scholarly work on contemporary issues related to bioethics, humanism, and professionalism in the Arab World (http://www.aub.edu.lb/fm/shbpp/Pages/index.aspx).

In dealing with bioethical issues, major Muslim countries have developed legal instruments.

For instance, in some countries, parliaments have passed bioethics-related legislation or relevant government authorities have codified bioethical norms, guidelines, or recommendations. In this regard, it is noteworthy that there are national bioethical codes in medical research as well as organ transplantation laws in Islamic countries such as Iran, Saudi Arabia, Turkey, and Pakistan.

In Iran, for example, the Organ Transplant Act was passed by Parliament in 2000, the Act of Embryo Donation to Infertile Spouses was ratified by Parliament in 2003 and the Therapeutic Abortion Act was passed by Parliament in 2005 (Bagheri 2014). The National Ethical Codes in Biomedical Research and the Patient's Charter of Rights were incorporated into regulation by the Ministry of Health through an administrative order. In Lebanon, the Code of Medical Ethics has a charter of law which was established in 1994 (Code of Medical Ethics, 1994). In Turkey, the Grand National Assembly has ratified several international bioethics conventions by such as the Convention on Human Rights and Biomedicine and the UN Convention on the Elimination of all Forms of Discrimination against Women and the Rights of Children. The Law on Population Planning of 1983 allows abortion under certain conditions and is one of the first bioethical issues that is governed by the legislation (Arda 2014). The Turkish Organ and Tissue Transplantation Law (1979) governs issues related to organ removal and transplantation.

In Saudi Arabia the organ transplantation law allows organ removal from brain-dead patients for organ transplantation (Saudi Center for Organ Transplantation 2016).

In terms of available resources in Islamic bioethics, since 2012, the Islamic Medical and Scientific Ethics Database, which has been developed by Georgetown University in Qatar, covers bioethics literature written in Arabic, English, and Farsi. This collection provides a bridge for international reflection on bioethics. (http://guides.library.georgetown.edu/c.php?g=75873&p=489527).

Another initiative to provide a comprehensive collection of resources with bibliographic records related to Islamic bioethics in English is the Encyclopedia of Islamic Bioethics which will soon be published by Oxford University Press in 2017.

## Capacity Building in Islamic Bioethics

Islamic countries vary in terms of capacity building in bioethics. While there are countries like Saudi Arabia, Iran, and Turkey with very strong bioethics educational programs and fairly good institutional capacity to deal with ethical dilemmas in biomedicine, many Islamic countries lack the necessary capacity in bioethics. In a questionnaire survey among Muslim bioethicists, capacity building was listed as number four in the top ten bioethics challenges and priorities in Islamic bioethics (Bagheri 2014). However, it is worth mentioning that each Islamic country may have different bioethical priorities and challenges.

The current situation shows that in many Islamic countries the most progressive capacity has been built in ethics in research and bioethics committees. The initiatives taken by international organizations such as UNESCO and the World Health Organization (WHO) can explain why research ethics and bioethics committees have been more developed in Islamic countries (Beloucif and Ben Ammar 2016). For instance, UNESCO is the force behind the establishment of national bioethics committees in many countries around the world including Islamic countries. These committees function on a national level, take into account the local religious norms, and provide ethical guidance. It is more than a decade since UNESCO encouraged and helped many countries to not only establish their own national bioethics committees but also organize different educational programs such as Teacher Training Courses which have been organized in Iran, Saudi Arabia, Malaysia, Indonesia, Oman, and Kuwait (UNESCO 2017).

In terms of capacity, due to the importance of ethical standards in conducting biomedical research, especially in clinical trials, the WHO has encouraged and helped member states to build capacity in research ethics by establishing research ethics committees. Currently, almost all Islamic countries who have capacity in biomedical research also have established research ethics committees. Countries such as Saudi Arabia, Iran, Turkey, Indonesia, Malaysia, Pakistan, Oman, Qatar, and Tunisia have developed their own national ethical codes in biomedical research. Given the fact that Islamic bioethics is very engaged with Islamic jurisprudence, any progress in bioethical deliberation depends not only on building capacity in bioethics but also in juridical methodology. As observed by Abdulaziz Sachedina, "In general, ethical inquiry connected with moral epistemology or moral ontology is underdeveloped in the Muslim seminarian curriculum which is, in large measure, legal-oriented" (Sachedina 2009, 9).

For Islamic bioethics to be able to address and resolve highly controversial bioethical issues, it is also important to focus on the juridical methodology, and one should go beyond the *fatwa* literature to understand the legal reasoning behind it.

## Conclusion

There is an increasing interest in the West in understanding medical ethics from the Islamic perspective. Both Muslim and non-Muslim healthcare providers have shown a sustained interest in Islamic viewpoints in medical practice and research in order to better serve the healthcare needs of the Muslim population in western countries. However, to be able to address bioethical issues and dilemmas in the Islamic context, capacity building in Islamic bioethics is necessary.

In developing Islamic bioethics, the task should focus on the methodological approach in extracting ethical deliberations, resolving ethical dilemmas, and making necessary recommendations that can guide human action for healthcare providers, policy makers as well as the public at large. In terms of capacity building in Islamic bioethics, as emphasized by several Islamic scholars, Muslim bioethicists should develop their own bioethics frameworks based on native Islamic teachings, culture and Islamic values instead of just translating and mimicking western secular bioethics.

## References

Abu Abdallah Muhammad. 1002/393 AH. *Al-Mustadrak alaa al-Sahihain, Volume 2*. 282.

Albar, M. A. and Chamsi-Pasha, H. 2015. *Contemporary Bioethics Islamic Perspective*. New York: Springer.

Arda, B. *et al.* 2014. Bioethics in Turkey. In: ten Have and Gordijn (eds.). *Handbook of Global Bioethics*. New York: Springer.

Bagheri, A. and Afshar, L. 2011. Abortion in Different Islamic Jurisprudence: Case Commentaries. *Asian Bioethics Review*, Special Issue on Islamic Bioethics 3(4), 351–365.

Beloucif, S. and Ben Ammar, M. S. 2015. Bioethics in Arab Region and the Impact of the UNESCO International Bioethics. In: Bagheri, A. *et al.* (eds.). *Global Bioethics: The Impact of the UNESCO International Bioethics Committee*. New York: Springer.

Code of Medical Ethics in Lebanon. 1994. Law No. 288, 1994. Official Gazette 9. Beirut.

Hattab, A. S. and Ramon, A. J. 2004. Bioethics in the Arab World, the Experience of Aden Medical School. *Revista LatinoAmericana De Bioethica*. 1(1), 1–16.

Ragab, A. R. A. 2014. Bioethics in Egypt. In: ten Have and Gordijn (eds.). *Handbook of Global Bioethics*. New York: Springer.

Sachedina, A. 2009. *Islamic Biomedical Ethics, Principles and Application.* Oxford: Oxford University Press.

Sastrowijoto, S. *et al.* 2014. Bioethics in Indonesia. In: Ten Have and Gordijn (eds.). *Handbook of Global Bioethics.* New York: Springer.

Saudi Center for Organ Transplantation. 2016. Organ Transplantation in Saudi Arabia. Available at: http://www.scot.org.sa/eng-index.html. [Accessed December 1, 2016].

Shabana Ayman. 2013. Religious and Cultural Legitimacy of Bioethics: Lessons from Islamic Bioethics. *Medicine, Health Care and Philosophy* 16(4), 671–677.

Shapiro G., *et al.* (eds.). 2015. *Islamic Ethics of Life: Abortion, War and Euthanasia.* London: Koros Press.

Shomali, M. A. 2008. Islamic Bioethics: A General Scheme. *Journal of Medical Ethics and History of Medicine*, 1(1). Available at http://www.ncbi.nlm.nih.gov/pmc/articles/PMC3713653. [Accessed 15 December 2016].

Turkish Organ and Tissue Transplantation Law. 1979. Turkish Organ and Tissue Transplantation Code, No. 2238 (1979).

UNESCO Teacher Training Courses. Available at: http://www.unesco.org/new/en/social-and-human-sciences/themes/bioethics/ethics-education-programme/activities/ethics-teacher-training/. [Accessed January 2017].

# CHAPTER THREE

## What Islamic Bioethics Offers to Global Bioethics

*Alireza Bagheri, Alastair Campbell, Carol Taylor,*
*James Rusthoven, Jonathan Crane and Abdallah Daar*

### Summary

In the era of globalisation and multiculturalism, participation of Islamic bioethics in a dialogue with other religious-based bioethics is crucial. Such a dialogue within a rigorous examination of comparative religious ethics would help scholars in the field share their concerns as well as practical solutions for bioethical dilemmas.

This chapter presents five commentaries from renowned Muslim, Christian, and Jewish bioethicists responding to the question: what does Islamic bioethics offer to global bioethics? Each author thoughtfully examines this question based on his or her own cultural and religious background. Each commentary elaborates on the importance of Islamic bioethics in contemporary bioethics; how it contributes to global bioethics; what new concepts it offers; as well as what can be learned. This chapter provides a platform for a multi-faith bioethics dialogue with the aim of better understanding Islamic bioethics.

## Introduction

The ethical dilemmas posed by new advances in science and technology have challenged all societies, religious as well as non-religious alike.

While a few decades ago religion was the primary basis for resolving ethical dilemmas in biomedicine, the secularisation of bioethics has gained more popularity in bioethical discussions. As observed by Daniel Callahan, "… the field of bioethics has moved from one dominated by religious and medical tradition to one now increasingly shaped by philosophical and legal concepts" (Callahan 1990).

Currently, each society addresses bioethical challenges and dilemmas based on their socio-cultural background, referencing religious beliefs or, alternatively, natural moral law or reason in secular bioethics. In many religious societies, for example in Muslim countries, the religious tradition continues to be the dominant approach and the main source in responding to the ethical questions in biomedicine. However, in the era of western-dominated healthcare technologies, concerns have been raised that by importing new biotechnology from the West, one has to also adopt western bioethics. In fact, the concern about "cultural identity" is at the center of using western biotechnology with its attached value system. This became the main concern especially for people in Asia, Latin America, and Africa. For instance, it has been argued that "… the globalisation of western technology should not be accompanied by the globalisation of western ways of thinking and acting … other cultures should be able to beg, borrow or buy western technology without having to take it along with all its western packaging, its entire surrounding value system" (Tangwa 1999). In Islamic societies, in which patients are mostly bound to observe their faith — especially in healthcare decision-making — Islamic bioethics urges Muslim physicians as well as health policy makers to focus on religious-based solutions in dealing with ethical dilemmas in the application of new biotechnology. If, in a broad sense, one can categorize bioethics into religious and non-religious bioethics — as the mainstream global bioethical discussions — then the task of this chapter is to see how Islamic bioethics can contribute to religious bioethics as well as to non-religious bioethics.

In comparing religious and secular bioethics Robert Veatch observes that: "… for those whose ethics has a religious base, their foundation is the will of the deity or his or her judgment of moral approval. To the extent that their theology is monotheistic, they must believe in a single grounding of moral judgment — God." Therefore, Islamic bioethics shares substantial common ground with other divine religions. Moreover, such common ground seems recognisable even to non-religious bioethics as well. Veatch also argues that, "Likewise, secular universalism holds there is some single grounding: the natural moral law, the dictates of reason, or some common morality shared by all reasonable people" (Veatch 1999). Therefore, in today's pluralistic and multicultural world, Islamic bioethics with its capabilities can become a conversation partner in bioethical debates with scholars in other religious as well as non-religious traditions of ethical reflection. This brings not only an opportunity to learn from other bioethical systems but also to offer some innovative approaches in dealing with bioethical issues.

The following elaborates on some characteristics of Islamic bioethics and the areas that Islamic bioethics can offer and learn from other bioethics value systems.

## Bioethics and Religion

An important debate has been taking place in bioethics literature: should bioethics take religion into account or is "irreligious bioethics" preferred? In defence of irreligious bioethics, Timothy (2012) has argued that: "Irreligious skepticism toward religious views about biomedical issues can yield important benefits to the field ... bioethics needs a vigorous irreligious outlook every bit as much as it needs descriptive understandings of religion."

In fact, at least in religious societies, in which people rely on religious norms in healthcare decision-making, appealing to irreligious bioethics risks an alienation of bioethics in that society. The fact that religion is well-represented in bioethical debates is evident by the immense volume of publications that address religious perspectives in bioethical issues.

No matter how forceful the argument for a religiously-neutral bioethic, the fact remains that the only way for many people to deliberate and resolve serious bioethical problems is to appeal to religion (Shabana 2013). This can be an important message from Islamic bioethics to global bioethics that while many people around the world rely on their faiths to resolve bioethical dilemmas not only in their private, individual healthcare decision-making but also in the broader bioethics-related public policy-making, an irreligious bioethics or a religiously-neutral bioethics would fail in its applicability on a global scale.

### Existing collaboration between Islamic jurists, physicians and scientists

In practice, there is a constructive collaboration between Islamic jurists as the "experts of the texts" and scientists as the "experts of the context" to provide ethical guidelines for such complex dilemmas. For instance in the case of emerging issues such as organ removal from dead brains, stem cell research, and assisted reproductive technologies, a set process is followed to find solutions. First, a physician, or a group of physicians, who face an ethical dilemma in their practice seek to find a religious opinion by explaining the problem to an Islamic jurist (*faqih*) or to a committee of Islamic scholars. In case of approval by the religious authority, the issue is taken to the health authority for the development of national guidelines or to the parliament for policy-making, as needed. This procedural approach ensures participation of all relevant stakeholders and a guarantee to the applicability of the suggested ethical resolution found through this process.

### Flexibility of Islamic bioethics

Compared to the individual rights-based Western bioethics, Islamic bio-ethics is a duty-based communitarian bioethics (Chamsi-Pasha and Albar 2014) which emphasizes the balance between individual rights and public interest. Islamic bioethics with its methodology is flexible to be able to accommodate public interests in its bioethics rulings.

In Islamic bioethics, deriving solutions for emerging bioethical dilemmas in medical practice and research can be accommodated by *Shari'a* as long as they are intended to benefit humanity. As observed by Farhat Moazam (2011), in Islamic bioethics "discussions and rulings are not fashioned in a vacuum but shaped by interplay of perceived boundaries of authority within political and legal systems and existing societal norms." Such flexibility which seriously takes the "context" into account is a key in the interpretation of the "Text" guided by achieving public good.

### The complexity of the relation between ethics, law and fiqh

In all ethical systems, religious or non-religious, the relationship between ethics and law is an important issue. However, in the Islamic context there is another crucial factor: Islamic jurisprudence or *fatwa*. This factor plays a great role in bioethics deliberation in Islamic societies. An international study published in 2014, listed top 10 ten bioethical challenges in Muslim countries. The first priority was to define the relationship between law, ethics and *fatwa* (Bagheri 2014). In Islamic bioethics as argued by Sachedina (2011), it is important to distinguish between a "legal–religious ruling" and an "ethical resolution." The importance of such a distinction is not limited to Islamic bioethics; rather, all religious-based bioethics deliberation should make sure to determine the moral underpinnings of religious duties. How this relationship is defined in Islamic bioethics can be an example for other faith-based bioethics. No doubt, a constructive global dialogue can help Islamic bioethics learn from other bioethics value systems. For instance the importance of public discourse in bioethics, which has been given less attention in Islamic societies, is a learning point.

In the following commentaries, five scholars examine what Islamic bioethics can offer to the global bioethics.

## The Global Significance of Islamic Bioethics

### *Alastair Campbell*

Christianity and Islam are clearly closely related to each other, not as siblings perhaps but, at the very least, as cousins, since they both have origins in monotheism, as does Judaism. Each of these religious traditions has its own history of evolution and reform but there remain strong family resemblances between them. They share a belief in one God and that moral requirements are based on obedience to God's will. It is these common features that have led to the description of all three as "Abrahamic religions," setting them apart from the very different forms of spirituality found in Hinduism and Buddhism, for example. Certainly the history of relationships between these "Abrahamic" faiths is not a universally positive one, being mired in discrimination, misrepresentation and — all too often — violence. But, if we can get past this dreadful legacy, we get a clearer picture of how Christian and Islamic approaches to bioethics relate to each other. In this short commentary, I shall first consider a basic (and ancient) question — what is the relationship between religion and ethics?

Then I shall consider the similarities and differences between Islamic and Christian approaches to bioethics. Finally, I shall refer to the global significance of Islamic bioethics.

## Religion and ethics

In the *Euthyphro* Socrates poses the question: "Is something good because God wills it? Or, does God will it because it is good?" This is a classic dilemma If we answer "yes" to the first part then we seem committed to accepting morally outrageous requirements if they are claimed to be God's will (slaughtering the "infidels," for example). If instead we say "yes" to the second, then we seem to make God subservient to our conception of what is moral. The similarities and differences between Christianity and Islam can be seen as related to different ways of facing this dilemma. In fact, what is really interesting here is that both traditions show a diversity of approaches to this central quandary.

Both traditions have what might be classed as "fundamentalist" groups within them. As "religions of the Book" (the Qur'an, the *Sunna* and the Bible), there is a strong imperative to look to scripture for answers to the puzzling and new questions raised by modern bioethics. But the key question is the *interpretation* of what is written in these ancient texts. For the fundamentalist there is nothing to debate — the answer is plain for all to see. But this position is hard to sustain, given the ancient written texts do not mention, for example, stem cell transplantation or germ line engineering. Who is to discern God's will in such cases? Scholarship and interpretation become quite crucial if the religious tradition is to have anything relevant to say about bioethical issues, whether to its own community of believers or to society as a whole. From this challenge comes a strong similarity between the two faith traditions: in any honest attempt to interpret religious faith for the modern world there is inevitably a range of views about what is right, or about what is truly God's will. Allowing scholarship to enter in means grasping firmly *both* horns of the *Euthyphro* dilemma, leads to no simple answers. Of course dogmatists in both traditions deny that this is so, but there is no possibility of ignoring the wide range of opinions on controversial topics expressed by Muslim and Christian scholars alike (see Aramesh 2009 and Moazam 2011 for clear accounts of this diversity in Islamic scholarship).

## Faith, law and ethics

On the other hand, we should not ignore the distinctiveness of the traditions, by seeking some kind of bland, syncretistic faith to keep everyone happy! The name "Islam" itself sums up the distinctiveness of the Muslim way of life — "submission to the will of God." To some extent this distinctiveness is captured in the religious practices of devout Muslims, such as daily prayer at fixed times, fasting, alms-giving and the pilgrimage to Mecca, but, from the point of view of bioethics, it is the Islamic approach to dealing with ethical questions that sets it apart. This can be described as *jurisprudential* in nature: specific questions are addressed to jurists, who then come up with judgments (*fiqh*), and subsequently such judgments may lead to a binding requirement (*fatwah*). There is really nothing similar to this in Christian approaches to bioethics. In Roman Catholicism there is an appeal to "natural law" (on such matters as reproduction for example), but such law, it is claimed, would be binding on all humans, not just on believers; and Protestantism has been deeply suspicious of this approach, seeing it as a dangerous challenge to the uniqueness of faith. Again, in Christianity sometimes there are binding requirements based on religious authority (for example, the *ex cathedra* pronouncements of the Pope, which Catholics are supposed to obey without question), but the Islamic development of *Shari'a* law is really quite different from this. As Moazam put it (*op. cit.,* 319) it is not "uniform and frozen in time," but instead is in a constant state of evolution and refinement as it faces contemporary challenges.

## Global significance

What then of the global significance of Islamic bioethics? There is considerable suspicion among secular bioethics scholars regarding religious approaches to the subject. This is quite understandable, given the many examples in several religious traditions of doctrinaire approaches and the consequent suppression of dissent. But it would be folly to ignore the fact that, for millions of people across the world, religious faith of whatever tradition is a powerful influence on both ethical belief and sustained commitment to the moral life. There are also many secular ideologies that can be just as oppressive as narrow and dogmatic approaches to religion.

So the distinctive approach of modern Islamic bioethics, with its flexible and constantly evolving attempts to relate religious tradition to contemporary issues, and so to offer practical guidance to the many million followers of Islam, surely has a great deal to offer to global bioethics.

Moreover, from a practical point of view, bioethics (at least in that aspect which deals with healthcare ethics) has to be related to the way that doctors, nurses and other healthcare professionals deal with the dilemmas their patients face. The idea that "one size fits all" in bioethics is a view that I have strongly opposed over the years, since it results in some kind of cultural imperialism by western philosophical approaches to the subject. In my presidential address to the Fourth World Congress of Bioethics in 1998 I argued against the "homogenisation" of global bioethics. Instead I made a plea for diversity of approaches, including religious ones:

> Global Bioethics must respect the whole diversity of world views of ethics, both religious and non-religious.... I would say that faith of some kind (not necessarily religious) is a feature of all ethical commitment. (Campbell 1999, 189).

Given the multicultural nature of modern societies, I would argue strongly that a welcoming of such diversity in moral views is an essential feature of all professional care. Specifically, only by respecting and understanding the Islamic approach to ethics can non-Muslim healthcare workers give adequate care to those for whom this faith is fundamental to their moral choices.

## Global Significance of Islamic Bioethics: A Roman Catholic Perspective

### Carol Taylor

In an introduction to bioethics, Dan Callahan (1995) identified the three foundational questions in bioethics:

— What kind of person ought I to be in order to live a moral life and make good ethical decisions?
— What are my duties and obligations to other individuals whose life and well-being may be affected by my actions?

— What do I owe the common good or the public interest, in my life as a member of society?

There are an estimated 1.6 billion Muslims (or 23% of the world's population), "making Islam the world's second-largest religious tradition after Christianity." It matters greatly how Islam directs these questions be answered.

The Pew Research Center's Forum on Religion and Public Life conducted a worldwide survey of Muslims involving more than 38,000 face-to-face interviews in over 80 languages. Findings included:

— In addition to the widespread conviction that there is only one God and that Muhammad is His Prophet, large percentages of Muslims around the world share other articles of faith, including beliefs in angels, heaven, hell, and fate (or predestination).

— While there is broad agreement on the core tenets of Islam, Muslims across the 39 countries and territories surveyed differed significantly in their levels of religious commitment, openness to multiple interpretations of their faith, and acceptance of various sects and movements.

— Muslims also hold widely differing views about many other aspects of their faith, including how important religion is to their lives, who counts as a Muslim and what practices are acceptable in Islam (Pew Forum on Religion and Public Life, 2012, 7).

I have often experienced the differences in Muslims' religious beliefs and practices while teaching Muslim students in the health professions. In the fall of 2014, I had the opportunity to teach the first course on spirituality and medicine at the American University in Beirut, Lebanon to 100 second year medical students. Each student wrote four essays and their writings reflected great diversity. Among the themes explored were the following:

— Reflect on the role religion/faith commitments play in your family members' lives as they deal with birth, aging, sickness, and, ultimately, death. In what ways do religion/faith commitments promote or constrain healing, wellness, good dying?

— Do you have personal experience where religion played a positive role in helping a patient respond to the challenges of injury, illness, and dying? Do you have personal experience where religion created conflicts because religious beliefs/teaching contradicted good medical practice?

— Each country is different. Major differences exist among countries with secular and religious cultures. Identify at least five ways Lebanon's religious culture is influencing health legislation. In your judgment are these promoting health outcomes? In what ways, if any, do you think health policy needs to change?

While some students coming from traditional religious traditions like Islamic, Christian, and others all respected and appreciated the role their religion played in directing their stance toward life, other students were quick to identify conflicts between religious teachings and good medical practice. The differences between those who categorized religion as life-affirming and those who focused on religion as life-denying were striking. Davis and Zoloft (1999) identify significant questions colored by religious beliefs, attitudes and values.

— What is the meaning of suffering in the context of human life and cosmic reality?
— How should we regard the physical body and its functions?
— What is the meaning and role of gender differences, sexuality, and reproduction?
— How are we to understand and respond to birth, aging, and death?
— What constitutes the self, and how is selfhood to be assessed?
— How are sin and moral culpability understood? What makes something sinful and how is sin relieved or absolved?
— What are the tradition's specific bioethical teachings? How authoritative are they, and who is regarded as their proper interpreter?

For both Roman Catholics and Muslims the questions of "how authoritative moral teachings are" and "who is regarded their proper interpreter" have critical importance. Since neither the Christian Scriptures nor the Qur'an directly address many of the questions raised by today's scientific and technological advances, the question of interpretation is central. Many thoughtful individuals struggle to resolve questions that arise in existential contexts. In both Islamic and Roman Catholic traditions there is a tension between deductive processes that begin analysis with absolute principles to work down to particular judgments, and inductive processes that start with the experience of people in particular circumstances to reach tentative conclusions about which principles are relevant. While many find comfort in absolute religious truths, others find this approach legalistic. Similarly, while many value an approach grounded in the dignity of humans, others find this approach relativistic.

The Catechism of the Catholic Church assigns to the Church the right "always and everywhere to announce moral principles, including those pertaining to the social order, and to make judgments on any human affairs to the extent that they are required by the fundamental rights of the human person or the salvation of souls" (Taylor 1994, 491). It recognizes the Roman Pontiff and bishops as "authentic teachers" endowed with the authority of Christ. Central to the Roman Catholic understanding of morality, however, is appreciation for the role that pastors, theologians, and all Christians and persons of good will play in teaching and applying Christian morality. This is linked to the conviction that "the Holy Spirit can use the humblest to enlighten the learned and those in the highest positions" (Taylor 1994, 492).

Valid sources of truth in the Roman Catholic tradition thus include the Magisterium of the Pastors of the Church, theologians, and the *sensus fidelium*, or the "sense of the faithful." This source of truth represents the combined beliefs, consciences and experiences of good and honest Catholics. It operates in a close relationship of mutual conditioning with all of the other varied components of the Roman Catholic tradition. *Sensus fidelium* is, however, a disputed concept within the Church. The Catholic Theological Society of America made it the theme of its 70th annual convention in 2015 on the 50th anniversary of the closing of the Second Vatican Council. Among the questions they posed in their call for proposal were the following:

— How does the *sensus fidelium* serve as an impetus for the development of doctrine and the recognition and reception of the faith of the church?
— What is the role of the *sensus fidelium* in fundamental moral theology and in particular areas, such as, sexual ethics, human rights, poverty and economics, and war and peace?

— How are differences based on race, ethnicity, religious beliefs, and sexual orientation understood and negotiated in light of the category of the *sensus fidelium?*

— What is the relationship between the *sensus fidelium*, consensus, dissensus, differentiated consensus, public opinion, and common sense? http://www.ctsa-online.org/

Noting the absence of a central authority for all schools of thought in Islam, Bagheri (2014) sees "a constructive collaboration between Islamic jurists as the experts of the texts and scientists as the experts of contexts to provide ethical guidelines for complex dilemmas (Bagheri 2014, 394). In his 2014 study, Islamic ethics experts ranked the relation between law, ethics, and *fatwa* (the opinion of qualified scholars of Islamic *Shari'a*) the number one priority among the 20 bioethical challenges in Islamic countries. At the very least, this seems to suggest that respectful hearing of one another and willingness to presume the good will and intention of the other matters greatly. The recent emphasis on the virtue of mercy in Roman Catholicism suggests that both deductive and inductive thinkers would benefit from careful discernment about mercy's role in ethical decision-making. Both Cardinal Kasper's book on mercy and Pope Francis' call for a Holy Year of Mercy recommend a non-judging, non-condemning church. I am reminded of the 2014 movie *Timbuktu* where the local imam, who is committed to upholding the existing traditions of a benevolent and tolerant Islam, repeatedly questions Islamic zealots who are using the Qur'an to support questionable behavior, "Where is the mercy? Where is the mercy?" It seems clear that wise and good persons in all religious traditions will need to continue to discern what kind of persons we ought to be in order to live a moral life and make good ethical decisions.

## Islamic Bioethics and What It Brings to Global Bioethics

### *James Rusthoven*

Bioethics initially developed as a contemporary discipline from a diversity of scholars and caregivers of various faith traditions. In efforts to develop a common language and common basic principles for the multi-cultural and multi-religious societal communities developing in Western countries, principles-based ethics became the dominant paradigm for discourse and decision-making in the discipline. However, over time, the importance and inclusion of religious beliefs as grounding for bioethical decisions and policies faded from importance, if not relevance, along with many bioethicists espousing those beliefs. In recent years the importance of such beliefs has gained increased recognition and the impact of religious belief on bioethical decision-making is becoming more openly discussed in public debate.

In April 2011, I was given the privilege of attending the conference "Where Religion, Policy, and Bioethics Meet: An Interdisciplinary Conference on Islamic Bioethics and End-of-Life Care" as the representative of the Canadian Council of Churches. The conference was held to address Muslim concerns over the formation of an Islamic bioethics by Muslims and brought together views of Muslim caregivers and scholars from around the world. For a Christian with an advanced knowledge of the history of struggles within my own religious tradition, the conference more widely opened my eyes to the impact of major differences within Islam on caring for patients at the end-of-life and understanding decision-making within different Islamic traditions. Key messages that I took away from the conference included a conscious struggle by influential Muslim scholars to work out whether those practicing Islam in medicine should use principles-based ethics as their bioethical framework or develop a uniquely Islamic bioethics. Another key message was that, like other Abrahamic faith traditions, Islam needs to contend with bioethical issues through an Islamic hermeneutic that draws from the Islamic faith in forming Islamic views on these issues. Also encouraged was interfaith collaboration within and across Islamic denominations as well as dialogue across Abrahamic faith traditions in relation to common threads of belief. At the end of the conference, I found myself in awe of the immense task before the Islamic faith community. As I began to see parallels with the history of the Christian tradition, I realized that their struggles are our struggles. At the heart of intra-faith differences in both faith traditions is the interpretation of written Word, coloured by the historical and cultural contexts within which its people of faith live. Yet the people of Islam seem to be under greater immediate pressure to work out their intra-faith differences between *Sunni* and *Shii'te* traditions as well as the major differences within those sub-traditions. This could be due to the longer history of theological differentiation in Christianity, particularly Protestant denominations. Nonetheless, I found striking parallels between the greater reliance of decision-making on theological grounds in *Shi'a* Islam and in Eastern Orthodox Christianity compared to the more legally grounded decision-making of *Sunni* scholars and jurists, and the greater emphasis on law and rationality in western Christian traditions.

Top bioethical challenges among Muslim countries have been identified (Bagheri 2014). Through careful reflection and the development of solutions grounded in the Islamic faith, Muslims can make formative contributions to bioethics globally. One of the most important contributions would be to develop an Islamic framework that intentionally embeds Islamic teaching and faith into bioethical decision-making. As noted earlier, Muslim leaders should decide if the principles developed in the West are also valid for Islamic caregivers and patients; whether other principles should be considered to replace, or to be added to, these principles; and whether the Islamic faith should lead to a particular moral framework distinct from that of principles-based ethics. Such work would be most helpful to other communities whose particular moral beliefs beg to understand bioethics as ethics beyond a minimal, common morality model.

A second major contribution of Islamic bioethicists to global bioethics can come in the articulation of how streams of faith traditions within the distinct denominations of Islam directly influence bioethical thinking, policy-making, and decision-making. What is the role of religious law and specific theological beliefs in end-of life decisions? How do they complement the contributions of different caregivers or create tensions among caregivers who do not share such basic beliefs when caring for a particular patient? How do Islamic medical communities of mixed Islamic beliefs resolve, or live with, their differences to the betterment of their patients, their communities, and society at large?

A third major contribution would be in the area of defining human rights and dignity. The liberal worldview out of which principlism developed prizes autonomy of the individual above the influence of basic beliefs of a particular collective group. As such, the concepts of human rights and dignity are defined by what is best for the individual and by the individual. Many adhering to Christian traditions struggle to overcome this view in working out concrete expressions of their particular Christian beliefs as we work in bioethics.

Islam, Christianity, and Judaism can enrich each other's faith tradition through understanding the struggles and insights of the others and by sharing these basic concerns while developing more overt and meaningful expressions of faith within bioethics, and working with common theological and relational themes such as covenantal-relating. We should also be encouraged by the publication of recent collaborative work resulting from dialogue between Reformed Christians and Muslims regarding common concerns over the risks of the globalization of technology on the created order (Jochemsen and van der Stoep 2010). Challenges to the social and ethical fabric of faith communities will continue to grow in our rapidly changing world as brought about by new technologies and allied cultural changes. Islam can teach lessons of reflection and wisdom in response to the growing challenges within medical practice and research. Not only Christianity and Judaism, but any tradition of faith can learn from such wisdom and enrich their own struggles in their confrontation with the ethical and social challenges of bioethics in the 21st century.

## Global Significance of Islamic Bioethics: A Jewish Perspective

### *Jonathan Crane*

The modern Jewish philosopher Lenn E. Goodman (2008) writes of "an on-going dialectic between ethics and religion, as our insights about value, including moral value, inform and are informed by our ideas of the divine. This is the dialectic I call 'chimneying,' borrowing the image from the climbers who push off opposing rock faces as they work their way upward in a narrow defile." Such chimneying between ideals and ideas, what ought to be and what is, — ethics and law, divine revelation and human reason — is an enterprise common to both Islamic and Jewish bioethics. The preeminent Islamic bioethicist Abdulaziz Sachedina, an old friend of Goodman's, similarly speaks of chimneying, of "moving back and forth between juridical and ethical traditions in Islam" (Sachedina 2009, 12). In his view, the search for a paradigm case that could guide bioethical decision-making moves back and forth from normative to present case, from history to modernity. The resolution in the legal case is the *ḥukm*, which carries the authority of being implemented, whereas the resolution in the ethical case is a provisional conclusion to provide a recommendation that could change as the case begins to unfold in its complexity, seeking a justifiable course of action (Sachedina 2009, 21). In this way, practice (*mu'āmalāt*) is distinct from guidance (*mu'ābarāt*), with law predominating in the former and ethics the latter. Bounding between these edifices is what Islamic bioethicists do.

The solidity of these edifices is simultaneously given and questionable. On the one hand, Islamic law — *Shari'a* — is understood to be divine revelation, pertinent to all aspects of human existence and conduct, and geared toward perfecting humans toward salvation. It is a solid and broad rock upon which all acts are classified into such categories as the incumbent or compulsory (*wājib*), the recommended (*mustahabb*), the permitted or free (*mubāh*), the disapproved or reprehensible or unadvised (*makrūh*), and the forbidden (*ḥarām*). Once situated, an act cannot be relocated or reclassified, except in extremely limited and dire circumstances.

This raises the other hand: some *novums* arise, like new technologies or opportunities especially in medicine and scientific research that, though not dire, are nonetheless so strange that they cannot be readily classified according to the tried and true jurisprudential reasoning that has developed in Islamic communities over the past several centuries. Figuring out whether they are necessary, good, or evil, is no easy task. Some, like the *Ash'arites* and most *Sunnis*, hold that things and acts are good or evil precisely because God stipulated them so: those that are obligatory are good, those that are prohibited are evil.[1] Definability — can an act be classified one way or the other — is the exercise. Others, like the *Mu'tazilites* and *Shi'ites*, contend that God's command or prohibition is irrelevant to whether an act or thing is good or evil. Its essence, category and circumstance matter more than divine utterance. Defensibility — can an act be reasonably justified — is thus open for debate. On this account, agent morality is of paramount concern, whereas act morality is more central to the other groups.

---

[1] This obviously echoes Socrates' question about the relationship between the gods and the good. See Plato's *Euthyphro*, 10a.

It is thus all but impossible to speak of Islamic bioethics as a uniform and unvariegated discipline (Atighetchi 2007). Islamic scholars and jurists contribute to bioethical conversations from their preferred vantage points. Some lean heavily upon revelation and law, others more upon reason and ethics. A creative dynamic thus appears in the literature in which the inter-relationships between law, reason, revelation, and ethics are at issue — a conversation also afoot amongst Jewish bioethicists. Unsurprising, then, is the finding that the most pressing concern for Islamic bioethicists is the relation between law, ethics, and judicial (*fatwa*) opinion (Bagheri 2014). Indeed, methodological and procedural concerns predominate their top concerns: justice and health resource allocation; human rights; bioethics capacity building; patient's rights; Islamic principles of bioethics; bioethics committees — to name a few of the top ten. If the heady issues of balancing law and ethics, allocating powers and clarifying principles are of greatest concern, it means that more earthy and fleshly issues are perceived to be less pressing, such as beginning of life issues and interventions, women's health ethics, environmental ethics, nanoethics. It will probably be the case that as technologies advances in the latter basket of issues, more attention will be given to them even though the heady issues remain unconcluded.

The global significance of Islamic bioethics as a field rests less in what it thus far has articulated on specific technology or case. Rather, its contribution will be in how Islamic bioethicists continue to think deeply about the ongoing (eternal?) procedural connections between reason and revelation, between ethics and law, while at the same time addressing the pressing issues of lived life. As patients transcend national and communal boundaries with the rise of healthcare tourism; as doctors go on missions to serve in distressed communities; as infectious diseases recognize no boundaries whatsoever; as technologies quickly spread, the global need for thoughtful and timely Islamic bioethical discourse is only increasing.

## What Islamic Bioethics Can Offer to Global Bioethics

### Abdallah Daar

Islam is not monolithic for it shares much with other western monotheistic religions. Every major religion has the characteristics of its own.

Fundamentally what is shared in all religions is a belief in the sanctity of life. In the Qur'an, the same verse that forbids taking life also promotes and urges the use of reason "This has He instructed you that you may use reason" (6: 151). In this brief commentary, which can only come from a personal perspective, I will focus on a few generalizable, interconnected issues based on my experience of bioethics as largely applied to global health and to new technologies. I focus on those aspects that have been *emphasized* perhaps more in Islam, recognizing that they may not all be exclusive to Islam.

In Islam there is complete resonance between religion and science such that it is incomprehensible to an understanding Muslim to be told that certain scientifically proven realities are anti-Islamic or anti-religion. In my reading, even Darwinian evolution, sometimes a controversial subject to Muslims, is Islamic. There are traces of evolutionary theory in Islamic discourse way before Darwin was born. There are even those who have argued that Darwin himself might have been influenced by Islamic thinkers (Shah 2015). There is no contradiction for believers in accepting that Allah's intention in creating new species may unfold through the very mechanisms of molecular evolution.

Along the same lines of thinking, there really is no distinction between "nature" and anything else — to a believer all are signs of creation and divine intent. What then of the role of humans? They are vicegerents of Allah on earth — i.e. Allah's representatives on earth, those who fulfil Allah's functions of creation, protection, and preservation here on earth. Humans are the guardians of God's creation (Nasr 2015). This realization, of course, comes with huge responsibilities: not only to leave behind a better place; to think seriously of the impact of our current actions on future generations; and also to take stewardship of the environment, here and now, very seriously indeed. This of course includes addressing climate change, a point made very well in the recently released Islamic Declaration on Global Climate Change (2015).

Although hardly excelling in higher education today (Guessoum and Osama 2015), Muslims do take seriously the imperative to seek knowledge. This means not only being open to new discoveries by others, but to seek new knowledge in terms of research and letting the evidence lead to whatever conclusion. An opportunity for Muslim societies is to invest in serious scholarly work while raising the standards of education all the way from primary education to the highest levels of higher education. In this respect, for some, oil wealth has truly been a setback and a curse because it has eroded the hunger for knowledge and the need for creativity. The challenge then is to be at the forefront of change based on evidence, rather than simply being consumers of scientific discoveries made elsewhere.

Faith, reason, and rationality coexist solidly in Islam. In my view, the most highly evolved organ in the known universe, certainly here on earth, is the human brain. I would argue that always looking back to past guideposts through the dimness of time instead of using that organ to the maximum extent is an enormous and dangerous waste — perchance even the greatest sin. This is not the time to be led by past and present certainties. Reflection means starting with an open question and mind, starting with a doubt that you seriously, genuinely, objectively chip away at until you glimpse the truth. Islam appeals to the intellect.

The lack of emphasis on miracles in Islam can only mean that the fundamental laws of the universe — be they the laws of physics, chemistry or biology — are unimpeachable. On this earth, two plus two will always be four. Hiding behind the notion that certain realities are inexplicable to us because they are God's secrets (and this notion is sometimes used as an argument for the existence of God) leads to a mentality of fatalism, inaction and lack of responsibility. Fatalism has no place in Islam. One of the greatest challenges facing humankind today is the over-consumption of resources, degradation of the environment, threats to biodiversity, and climate change. Taking our stewardship responsibilities seriously, therefore, is vital. We should not shrug in the face of large challenges, holding that God has decreed these challenges and there is nothing we can do about them. If we adopt this attitude then we increase the threats to our lives and to those of future generations. Stewardship of the environment is intimately linked to the belief in the sanctity of human life and the necessity to protect life on earth.

Muslims greet each other with a salutation containing the word *salaam*: peace. Perhaps more than in any other religion this aspiration to peace is a constant reality. Without peace there can be no development, no health, and no human thriving (or indeed animal and plant life). How is it then that we have so little peace today around the world? Think of the Congo,

South Sudan, Ukraine, and indeed of many parts where Muslims live, particularly in the Middle East. Our tendency to explain this lack of peace as a result of, justifiably, the historical role of colonialism (and of our own past errors) will not help to solve all our problems in the future. Rather than inclining us to emphasize the differences, history teaches us of the aimlessness and nihilism of conflict and war. The Qur'an teaches us to respect one another and live in peace (3:64). Pluralism is in the DNA of Islam. So what is yet another Muslim emphasis to get us out of this morass of lack of peace? That emphasis might well start with the governance concept of *shura*: in reality creating truly open civil spaces wherein serious conversations are not dominated by the elite or the violent. Participation in civil discourse is also reflected in the emerging ethical principle of community engagement, especially in global health research (Tindana *et al.* 2015). The inability to listen is one of our greatest deficiencies as humans. Yet, to survive and thrive, we must learn to listen — with humility and objectivity, both of which are better served with prior reliable information — hence the emphasis on seeking knowledge.

The idea of humans as Allah's vicegerents on earth also means not fearing new technologies whether applied to health, personal improvement, the environment, or the rest of creation around us, including other animals. Technologies as such are not evil but their application can be evil, as with the misuse of nuclear power. We must therefore be open to creating and accepting new technologies — but our stewardship responsibilities require that we must think about ethical applications, and that means smart regulations (not just rules, but resources and tools for the implementation of those rules). Women in Islam were amongst the first, if not the first, systematically to acquire real civil rights, including those of property ownership independent of men. There is no place for gender inequality in Islam. If we find it, we must work hard to eliminate it so that women can take their rightful place amongst policy-makers and leaders. That must begin with equal, high-quality, education for girls and boys alike — and the total avoidance of stereotyping women as the weaker sex needing protection by men. The sad situation of women today in some parts of the developing world is largely due to the fact that men make all the important decisions.

Muslims do not subscribe to the idea that certain peoples are "chosen" in any way, including having special responsibilities, or that some are intrinsically better than others. No one is "chosen." We are all chosen if we wish to choose. Islam is colorblind. To Muslims #blacklivesmatter has always been a reality (http://blacklivesmatter.com). We are invited to regard differences as blessings, and to see tribes not as barriers between us but as a way to recognize and know one another. The "favored" are those who truly aspire to be close to God. This universalistic outlook of Islam is a true blessing if we internalize it deeply. Fortunately, it has been greatly emphasized, but it needs more emphasis in the future. It is also important to go beyond our respect and care only of the Western monotheistic religions, and encompass the Eastern religions, Hinduism, Buddhism, Jainism, Taoism, etc. in our ambit of sisterhood and brotherhood. The challenge of the time is to rise above and beyond narrow, parochial, tribal, obscurantist understandings and interpretations of Islam, and truly encompass the universalism deeply rooted in Islam. If we truly understand God's omnipotence, then it is incumbent on us to live in peace with adherents of all religions, else we doubt God's omnipotence: if God wanted to, could God not make all peoples Muslims? As it reads, "And had your Lord willed, those on earth would have believed — all of them entirely" (10:99).

There must be a Godly reason for that not being so. Or perhaps to Allah the definition of a Muslim extends way beyond what we think it is. The imperative to help others, to reduce poverty, and to reduce inequities is built into the fabric of Islam — most visibly through the institution of tithing (*zakaat*), wherein we are called to share part of our wealth with others in the service of Allah. And since Allah needs nothing from us — we are called to serve those, all those, that we can help. What needs to be emphasized more here is sustainability — we ought to use the important public institution of *zakaat* to empower people whenever possible, to avoid dependencies and their resulting humiliations. Compassion and solidarity ought to go beyond the sharing of money. Within the Qur'an and *hadith* and in the determinations of enlightened jurists, Islam has an overarching drive towards an ethical life (Daar and Khitamy 2001). Choice and responsibility underlie Islam, not the rituals. An ethical life is not to be constrained solely by past human encumbrances, including juridical decisions — for anything human-made is itself necessarily constrained by a worldview, an understanding, a certain way of reasoning, a personal history, and other human failings. Those human decisions and determinations need to be revisited and re-interpreted when necessary. An ethical life must be an examined life. Islam rose to its highest peaks when paired with critical thinking. We must truly understand what it means to be an exalted member of the human species, with responsibilities to other creatures and to this small, constrained biosphere.

## References

Aramesh, K. 2009. Iran's Experience on Religious Bioethics: An Overview. *Asian Bioethics Review* 1(4), 318–328.

Bagherie, A. 2014. Priority Setting in Islamic Bioethics: Top 10 Bioethical Challenges in Islamic countries. *Asian Bioethics Review* 6(4), 391–401.

Brockopp, J. E. (2008) Islam and Bioethics: Beyond Abortion and Euthanasia. *Journal of Religious Ethics*, 36(1), 3–12.

Campbell, A. V. 1999. Global Bioethics: Dream or Nightmare? *Bioethics* 13(3/4), 183–90.

Callahan, D. 1990. Religion and Secularization of Bioethics. *Hasting Center Report* 20(4), 2–4.

Callahan, D. 1995. Bioethics. In: Reich, W. T. (ed.). *Encyclopedia of Bioethics*, Rev. ed. New York: Macmillan Library Reference, 247–56.

Daar, A. S. and Khitamy, A. 2001. Bioethics for Clinicians: 21. Islamic Bioethics. *Canadian Medical Association Journal* 164(1), 60–3.

Atighetchi, D. 2007. *Islamic Bioethics: Problems and Perspectives.* Dordrecht, The Netherlands: Springer.

Davis, D. S. and Zoloth, L. 1999. *Notes from a Narrow Ridge: Religion and Bioethics.* Hagerstown, MD: University Publishing Group.

Islamic Declaration on Global Climate Change. 2015. Available at http://islamicclimatedeclaration.org/islamic-declaration-on-global-climate-change/. [Accessed Nov 16, 2015].

Jochemsen, H. and van der Stoep, J. (eds.). 2010. *Different Cultures — One World: Dialogue Between Christians and Muslims About Globalizing Technology.* Amsterdam: Rozenberg Publishers.

Kasper, W. 2014. *Mercy: The Essence of the Gospel and the Key to Christian Life.* Mahwah, NJ: Paulist Press.

Goodman, L. E. 2008. *Love Thy Neighbor as Thyself.* New York: Oxford University Press, vii.

Moazam, F. 2011. Shariah Law and Transplantation: Through the Lens of Muslim Jurists. *Asian Bioethics Review* 3(4), 316–32.

Nasr, S. H. A. 2015. Religious Nature: Philosopher Seyyed Hossein Nasr on Islam and the Environment. *Bulletin of the Etomic Sciences* 71(5). Available at http://thebulletin.org/2015/september/religious-nature-philosopher-seyyed-hossein-nasr-islam-and-environment8721. [Accessed Nov 16, 2016].

Guessoum, N. and Osama, A. [Undated]. Institutions: Revive Universities of the Muslim World. Available at http://www.nature.com/news/institutions-revive-universities-of-the-muslim-world-1.18637 and http://muslim-science.com/science-at-universities-of-islamic-world-2/. [Accessed Nov 16, 2015].

Sachedina, A. 2009. *Islamic Biomedical Ethics: Principles and Application.* New York: Oxford University Press.

Shah, M. S. Pre-Darwinian Muslim Scholars' Views on Evolution. Available at http://pu.edu.pk/images/journal/uoc/PDF-FILES/(11)%20Dr.%20Sultan%20Shah_86_2.pdf. [Accessed Nov 16, 2016].

Taylor, Carol. 1994. English translation of the *Catechism of the Catholic Church* for the United States of America copyright © 1994, United States Catholic Conference, Inc. Libreria Editrice Vaticana.

Taylor, Carol. 2012. Pew Forum on Religion and Public Life: The World's Muslims: Unity and Diversity. Available at http://www.pewforum.org/Muslim/the-worlds-muslims-unity-and-diversity.aspx.

Tindana, P. *et al.* 2015. Community Engagement Strategies for Genomic Studies in Africa: A Review of the Literature. *BMC Medical Ethics* 16, 24.

# CHAPTER FOUR

## Gender and Sexuality in Islamic Bioethics

### *Ingrid Mattson*

### Summary

This chapter examines how various Islamic discourses assert and challenge normative claims about gender and sexuality. In the limited space assigned for this chapter, a comprehensive examination of these issues is impossible. Instead, it focuses on what are, in my opinion, some of the key problematic assumptions, dominant (and dominating) paradigms and under-developed principles that are invoked in discussions of gender and sexuality as they pertain to Islamic bioethics. This will necessarily involve, at times, a historical examination of how particular legal concepts and structures developed.

## Gender and Authority in Islamic Bioethics

Gender and sexuality are vast, expansive topics and are obviously (or should be) pertinent to other bioethical issues addressed in this book. For example: in evaluating doctor–patient relationships, concerns such as gendered authority; sexual versus clinical touching; and family paternalism must be addressed in the practice of medicine. Outside the clinic, in the seminaries and universities where theological assumptions and methodologies of Islamic bioethics are taught and evaluated, views about gender and sexuality will widely vary depending on the school of thought.

57

It is not only the curriculum, but the presence or absence of women along-side of men in teaching circles, mosques, seminaries, universities, and medical schools of each stream of thought that has a tremendous impact on how ethical knowledge is shaped and textured by local culture, shared anecdotes, and personal and group-gendered interests. Many of the major bioethical issues today — abortion, fertility, male and female circumcision, cosmetic surgery, adoption and surrogacy — relate directly to gender and sexuality. Despite this, works on Islamic bioethics by Muslim scholars display a remarkable lack of interest or urgency in involving all genders in any significant way in the decision-making process. And there is no indication in Muslim majority countries, where it is common for national policies on these issues to be decided by committees of religious scholars and scientific experts, that even a minimum of representation by women is required. Given the absence of legal protections for freedom of conscience and academic freedom in many Muslim majority countries, it is unrealistic to expect councils to articulate the experiences and needs of women, much less individuals who do not fit into rigid heteronormative and binary-gender presentations. While Abdulaziz Sachedina does not pay much attention to the lack of gender diversity in these bodies, he (2009, 12) notes the stifling context for most Islamic bioethics debates: "In the absence of consensual politics in the majority Muslim countries, healthcare policies are, in large measure, formulated without public debate over proper assessment of Islamic moral and cultural resources and without respect of human dignity and accruing human rights in furthering public and private health."

Many scholars privilege *fatwas* when researching Islamic bioethics. Rispler-Chaim (1993, 4) says that one of the greatest advantages of *fatwas* as a source for Islamic medical ethics "is that it assumes a dialogue between lay people and scholars." In this way, *fatwas* can be seen as a reflection of the needs and concerns of ordinary Muslims, integrated with the responses of scholars. One of the main limitations with researching bioethics through *fatwas*, Rispler-Chaim admits, is that only a limited number are published. It is therefore questionable how representative they are of the judicial opinions obtained by Muslims. It has been my experience in public settings that religious scholars will simply not respond to questions they deem too sensitive, controversial, or distasteful. More problematic, in my opinion, is that we cannot deduce how representative the published *fatwas* are of the most pressing concerns of ordinary believers. In addition, *fatwas* normally answer a narrow question and do not address all the relevant and particular concerns in a case. For example, Rispler-Chaim (1993, 7) comments on *fatwas* about abortion on which she was consulted: "Since questions pertaining to the legitimacy/morality of abortions are presented to religious figures and not to the physicians who perform abortions, there is obviously no interest in the surgical procedure itself, nor in its impact upon the woman's health or her future pregnancies. The only question is whether the *Sharī'a* is supportive of the operation or not."

In his study of traditional Islamic legal reasoning, Bernard Weiss (1998, 113) says that "the authority of jurists in Islam is an exclusively declarative authority," meaning that, unless these jurists are given a political or judicial appointment, in theory it is not obligatory for believers to comply with their decisions. Many Muslims, nevertheless, bind themselves to the rulings of particular scholars because of voluntary allegiance, social pressure, or an inability to access other opinions. In a country where Islam is declared the source or one of the sources, of law, there is a strong positivist quality to Islamic law (*fiqh*) as experienced by the people living in those countries. This is a consequence, in part, of the modern expansion of the traditional right of a Muslim government to enact regulations that are in accordance with the goals and limits of the law as established by religious scholars, a branch of Islamic constitutional law called *siyāsa shar'iyya*.[1] As Sachedina suggests, authoritarian political systems, to which many Muslims are subject, severely limit the possibility for citizens to participate in or challenge state policies and procedures. At the same time, large numbers of Muslims, even in authoritarian countries, reject and challenge official interpretations of the law. This is not a new phenomenon in Islamic societies, but one we have seen throughout history[2]; although evidence of such resistance in pre-modern times is often hard to locate, unless a notable person had taken a public stand. For contemporary societies, anthropological research, such as that undertaken by Morgan Clarke (2009) regarding reproductive technology in Lebanon, helps expand our understanding of the way Muslims engage with such *fatwas*. In our internet age it is easier than ever for a Muslim to follow the views of a scholar on the other side of the world, while rejecting, in conscience if not in practice, the official or dominant interpretations in the lands where they actually reside. Thus, determining what a majoritarian or a marginal position is among those who identify as Muslims, rather than that of published, government-sanctioned scholars, is not a simple task. Research always leaves an impact: distorting relationships, amplifying some authorities and diminishing others. When the opinions of well-known or state-sanctioned legal scholars are published as the current state of "Islamic bioethics," the views of many faithful Muslims who approach the same issues from different perspectives are marginalized. What is particularly salient in discussions about Islamic approaches to gender and sexuality in bioethics is the domination of the legal tradition by men. This does not mean that women have been absent from Islamic scholarship, even in the pre-modern period. Indeed, there is increasing evidence that Muslim women participated in many fields of religious scholarship throughout Islamic history in significant numbers.[3] However, women authorities have been hard to find among traditional legal scholars, much less among those who have held judicial power.

Nevertheless, as I have written elsewhere, even in the pre-modern era, "female authorities were never completely absent from the process of law-making and adjudication. Female witnesses were regularly called in paternity cases and in cases which required expertise in some aspect of female physiology or reproduction." Further, women "had opportunities to shape the law to the extent that custom was recognized by and incorporated into Islamic law. On matters on which revelation was silent, custom ('urf, 'adāt) was explicitly recognized as a source of law by the classical jurists.... What this means is that women were not simply passive recipients of legal rulings. Rather, where women had any power to shape and articulate community norms (a power that depended on a vast range of sociological and material factors) they had the ability to influence the application of the law (Mattson 2005a, 451)."

With modernity came the codification of the law which erased much of its diversity; separated "law" from individual spiritual guidance; and diminished the impact of the moral sentiments of a local community upon the law. Wael Hallaq (2009, 449–50) has demonstrated that the flexibility of pre-modern Islamic law came from a jurist's authority to draw upon the principles, concepts and opinions he considered most applicable to particular case. Codification, in contrast, which came from European example and pressure, "eliminates almost all such juristic and hermeneutical possibilities, leaving both the litigants and the judge with a single formulation and, in all likelihood, a single mode of judicial application." A "new patriarchy" arose out of nationalism which, Hallaq argues, "has always been a masculine conception that subordinates the feminine." Further, an "increasing sense of individualism, combined with a male-oriented national state, a new male-oriented economy and bureaucracy, and a wholesale collapse of the domestic economies that had been the exclusive domain of women, all combined to produce legal codes and legal cultures that, under the banner of modernity, tended to subordinate women rather than liberate them (Hallaq 2009, 458)." In this regard, a possible ethical issue which needs to be raised is whether the domination of men in most modern Islamic legal institutions creates an endemic conflict of interest on issues related to gender and sexuality.

Legal historians note that family law emerged from the colonial experience as "the preferential symbol of Islamic identity," placed in opposition to the West. The reality is that modern Islamic family law is not a pristine remnant of something "authentic," but is the result of accumulated social and political changes in the last few centuries that were then subject, particularly in neo-fundamentalist discourses, to a kind of arrested development. Kecia Ali (2016) clearly lays this out in her work on sexual ethics where she notes, for example, that concubinage was simply dropped out of modern works as if it never existed, while the underlying system of patriarchal control that traditional law gave to men over the sexuality of free and slave women was rarely addressed. Thus, this law, "which seemed to be the last fortress of the *Sharī'a* to survive the ravages of modernization (Hallaq 2009, 446)," was rather, a limb severed from the body of Muslim society.

The patriarchal impact of colonialism and fundamentalism has been ameliorated in many Muslim countries where women are increasingly present in public life as medical professionals, public officials, and religious scholars. Yet debates among Muslims over Islamic family law, which sets the parameters for discussions of Islamic bioethics related to gender and sexuality, are contentious, anguished, and far from resolved. Identity politics derail discussions of Islamic family law time and time again. What is "Islamic" is often negatively defined against what is seen as paradigmatically western. Shahidan (2008, 109) notes this dynamic in the medical literature of contemporary Iran, "When expedient the West is jettisoned as decadent and destructive, and imitating the West becomes reprehensible, yet the findings of the American Psychological Association are presented as objective proof for arguments without any qualification about the socio-historical context of psycho-physiological sciences."

In the internet age, spokespersons for various discursive streams of Islam — traditional, traditionalist, modernist, progressive, fundamentalist among others — vie for the hearts and minds of Muslims. The consequences of these schools' diverse approaches to Qur'anic hermeneutics, legal reasoning, and even cosmological doctrine are profound for their bioethical positions. If a particular school, for example, teaches that women and men are spiritually equal but that men have superior innate intellectual capacities and/or emotional regulation to women, they might teach that a female patient does not have the same bioethical right as a male to "autonomy". This paternalistic view of the relationship between men and women is commonplace in most traditionalist and fundamentalist schools of thought, but is challenged by progressive and feminist discourses.[4] Yet while almost all schools tolerate, in principle, juristic differences, the limits of toleration displayed by some are very narrow indeed with much of the male scholarly establishment rejecting any validity to feminist or progressive Qur'anic hermeneutics and deeming them to be Western innovations.

The conflation of Islam with patriarchal structures and a denial of female autonomy, with the latter deemed "western" constructs, is evident in this passage, taken from a book written by two Saudi medical professionals (Al-Bar and Chamsi-Pasha 2015, 109) about the "Islamic" approach to bioethics:

> *The western attitude of individualism is not accepted in many societies. In most countries of Asia, Africa, and the Middle East there is no health insurance for the public at large. Usually the family bears the burden of cost of any medical intervention.*
>
> *Similarly, there is no welfare state, and hence the breadwinner takes care of the elderly, the children, and ladies. Though females and children may be working at home, and in the field, or looking after the cattle and sheep of the family, they are usually not the breadwinners.*

*The role of the family and close friends should be respected in places where they have different philosophies and cultures that differ greatly from western liberal, individualistic patterns ... and health providers have to understand that there are different cultures that do not give priority to autonomy, as it is understood in the West.*

The concern for the extended family's role in providing financial support for dependent members in traditional societies has merit. Here, we see, perhaps, a legitimate attempt to address what Sachedina (2009, 28) criticizes as having happened thus far in wealthy Muslim nations such as Saudi Arabia where "advanced western medical technology is imported with little heed taken for its potential impacts on the political, economic, communal, social, and individual lives of the population." However, making agency and autonomy dependent upon whether one earns a wage is extremely problematic. Amina Wadud (2006, 142) notes that this "idealizes the woman as one who only reproduces and cares for offspring. Many assume that this is natural, and hence a voluntary contribution with no bearing on female agency." Further, the denial that women are "breadwinners" in "many societies" is a statement made without the support of any evidence, and in fact, seems more of an ideological stance in favor of traditional patriarchy.[5] In reality, what Bruce Caldwell (2006, 341) says about South Asian societies is true across much of the globe, "The population is rapidly urbanizing, thereby undermining the traditional patriarchal patrilineal families and beginning to offer choices to women other than marriage and childbearing, and enabling them to support themselves when abandoned without having to resort to socially unacceptable practices."

Those who wish to deny full autonomy (or less autonomy than men) to women in Islamic bioethics need to be clear about their reasons for doing so. And if those reasons depend not on claims about financial realities, which can be debated on the basis of facts, but on a scriptural hermeneutic that assigns men authority over women, then researchers need to know that there are alternative hermeneutics. Feminist, progressive, and egalitarian schools of Islamic thought are no less relevant to Islamic bioethics than traditionalist or fundamentalist schools of thought. Some argue "western influence" puts a culture in opposition to Islam (I do not believe it does). Given the increasing proliferation of western universities and medical institutions in wealthy Muslim countries, and coming in the wake of centuries of western colonialism and imperialism in many other countries, it is apparent that "westernization" is not confined to the Europe and the Americas. So-called "Muslim countries" are not necessarily, then, the best place to find an "authentic" or even widely-supported approach to Islamic bioethics. Among the most problematic aspects of many of these societies is the centralizing and homogenizing approach to Islamic law. As Asifa Quraishi (2010, 25) argues, "Muslim governments today are a deliberate departure from the pre-modern constitutional model that recognized a separation of *fiqh* and *siyasa* law [politics]. Instead, they are built on the nation-state model inherited from colonialism, where the government has a monopoly on all lawmaking power and there is no legally protected space for *fiqh* pluralism. When law is centralized in this way, these governments can easily be pressured to legislate and enforce one set of *fiqh* rules on everyone. This approach merges *fiqh* and *siyasa* power in a pseudo-theocratic way that was not possible in pre-modern systems." Some scholars, such as Faisal Rauf (2015), have even argued that the most "Islamic" discourses and views can be found, not in Muslim-majority countries, necessarily, but it in those societies where Muslims are free to challenge, express and debate legal opinions.

## Beyond Fiqh in Islamic Bioethics

The relevance of this reality to gender and authority in Islamic bioethics discourses today compels to include a greater plurality of Islamic hermeneutics and theological ethics, including feminist, progressive and egalitarian approaches in our surveys of Islamic bioethics. I submit that we also need to look beyond *fiqh* to other normative religious discourses if we are to argue for an "Islamic" perspective on bioethics, especially when it comes to seriously attending to the priorities and values of many Muslim women.

Guidance on bioethical issues is provided across the Muslim world not only by legal scholars and congregational imams, but by other authorities whose ranks include far more women than in the legal establishment: spiritual advisors (*Sufi sheikhs* among them), Muslim chaplains and respected elders. In these pastoral care and family settings, *fatwas* and other legal literature have a role, but they are not necessarily determinative of the guidance given. Key Islamic values such as mercy, forgiveness, and reconciliation, and the fundamental need to preserve faith in God come to the fore in these settings. More documentation of these encounters is needed to show the vital place of these values in the landscape of normative Islamic bioethics.

Islamic pastoral care is a developing field of religious authority critical to bioethics which draws upon the traditional legal and *Sufi* discourses.[6] Often such counseling helps the believer place a physical ailment in perspective such that she sees it as a positive opportunity for spiritual growth. For example, a woman might decide to eschew fertility treatment that has been deemed Islamically lawful in order to elevate her spiritual position by demonstrating trust in God (*tawwakul*). Can we say that we truly understand the landscape of Islamic bioethics if we marginalize such approaches? And if the preservation of a believer's relationship with God is prioritized in spiritual counseling, whether done on an informal or professional level, the most Islamic bioethical position in this context might be one which contradicts the law as commonly understood by people.

A number of Muslim feminists, such as Sa'diyya Shaikh (2015, 106–7), argue that some (not all) traditional *Sufi* teachings can help Muslims get past the "central deficits in various iterations of classical Islamic law" that are based in "limited gender understandings of human nature, as developed in different sociohistorical contexts." Shaikh says that "*Sufi* thinkers in particular have provided detailed discussions on the human condition; the spiritual landscape of human submission to the divine will; and the ways in which the fundamental theological imperative of submission provides the ontological basis for the juridico-ethical legacy and related norms of sociability." From a *Sufi* perspective, the law must be scrutinized to see whether our "understanding" (the literal meaning of *fiqh*) reflects the highest "religious and spiritual prerogatives in Islam."

This is not to argue that Islamic bioethics should be based in an antinomian "spiritual" hermeneutic. In most cases, Muslim counselors will still invoke a legal principle such as "necessity" to allow an individual exemption, rather than an outright contradiction, to the law. However, where advice is being given by spiritual advisors and among circles of family and friends, theological concepts such as God's mercy and forgiveness are, in addition to necessity, often articulated as legitimate Islamic grounds for veering from the law as asserted by scholars. These observations are anecdotal and without further research we cannot know whether Muslims view greater ethical or spiritual ends are being served when they put aside the law. They may not necessarily reject the law, but may believe that the scholars' legalistic understandings cannot be the whole picture. Nevertheless, the invocations of "necessity" and "mercy" are prodigiously used among Muslims to avoid legal judgments. Thus, the view that the dominant judgment of legal scholars is the correct Islamic one should be called into question.

## What "The Sleeping Child" Tells Us About the Priorities and Values of Islamic Ethics

As a case study, the adoption of "the sleeping child" phenomenon in early Islamic law demonstrates that the foundations for the principles underlying Islamic bioethics are less apparent than they might seem. The sleeping child phenomenon is reported to have been introduced into Islamic legal discourse at the earliest stage of its development, during the time of the second caliph, *'Umar ibn al-Khaṭṭāb* (ruled 634–644 AD). The situation that was presented to the caliph was that of a woman who had been widowed a few years earlier, then gave birth to a fully-developed baby only six months into her second marriage. As a result, the woman was suspected of having illicit relations before her current marriage and she faced negative consequences from various parties as a result. The caliph *'Umar* called for a midwife to serve as an expert witness to see if there was an explanation other than unlawful sexual relations for the woman's delivery of the full-term baby. The midwife testified that this was a case of a "sleeping child" (*al-raqīd*). She explained that the child's mother had been impregnated by her first husband but when he died, the baby was deprived of vital fluids due to the mother's extreme grief and had entered a state of hibernation. When the woman remarried, her new husband's seminal fluid reawakened the baby who then completed his development in six months. *'Umar* accepted this explanation by the female expert, thus rejecting claims that the atypical gestation period proved that the mother had illicit sex outside of marriage. The result was that the baby was deemed legitimate; had a right to inheritance and support from his "father's" estate and relatives; and the woman retained her reputation. The "sleeping child" phenomenon was integrated into the *Mālikī* school of law while other schools gave various alternative reasons to explain why a pregnancy could last much longer (up to five years) or shorter than usual (Mattson 2005, 450–1).

It was only at the turn of the 20th century, with the spread of western science and medicine, that these explanations were challenged by state-sanctioned legal authorities and secular medical authorities. Beginning in the 19th century, gender discourses were subject to "scientification," whereby folk medicine and "old wives' medicine" were criticized and derided as superstitious (El Shakry 2006, 345). "Starting in the 19th century and continuing until the present, a process of medicalization has transformed pregnancy and childbirth.... The displacement of traditional birth attendants by obstetricians and institution-trained midwives, surveillance of pregnancy by medical professionals, a shift in the location of childbirth from the home to institutional settings, and an increase in the number of obstetrical interventions characterize this process of medicalization (Stimler 2006, 342)." Certification in modern medicine depended on literacy which excluded many traditional healers, social classes and, in some places, for a certain period at least, women. Donna Lee Bowen notes that in the pre-modern period, the locus of most abortions was in homes, conducted through "popular medical practices," and that women "usually directly employed the remedies and conducted the procedures" despite the fact that medical and legal texts were written by men. In contrast, in contemporary Muslim societies, "The Islamic decision-making process which discusses permissibility of abortion is carried out by male jurists and scholars" (Bowen 2006, 314) and are conducted within a paternalistic, patriarchal medical system. It was in this context, the highly influential Egyptian modernist Muhammad Rashid Rida (d. 1935) was "troubled" by the contradiction between the duration of pregnancy as recognized by medicine and Islamic law and "wished to remove all differences between Muslim believers and scientific truth, hence he encouraged Muslims to embrace the findings of medicine (Rispler-Chaim 1993, 8)." In Morocco, where the "sleeping child" was firmly ensconced in the *Mālikī* legal tradition, this led to struggles over the authority of science to overturn traditional *Mālikī* law (Jansen 2000).

In dispensing with laws that allowed for shortened or lengthened gestational periods, it seems the modernists assumed that earlier jurists based laws on incorrect scientific theories simply because they did not know any better. This may be incorrect. If we consider the story of the law's origin under *Umar*, we could interpret it to mean that he was searching for a "way out" for the woman. After all, the fact that the people around her accused her of engaging in illicit sexual relations because of the child demonstrates that people in 7th century Arabia were well-aware of how long a full-term pregnancy lasted. Over the centuries, as the diverse schools of Islamic law developed their distinctive doctrines, it is striking that most of them accepted some theory of atypical pregnancy which would allow more children to be deemed legitimate. The Prophetic *hadith*, "The child belongs to the marriage bed," was interpreted by some scholars to mean that as long as a couple were married and the husband did not challenge the paternity of the child, the child was deemed legitimate; and for some scholars even in the case where the couple had been married only one month (Semerdjian 2008, 152). Clearly there was little eagerness on the part of jurists to sever the bonds of family and community in the service of scientific truth.

The continued reluctance of religious scholars in allowing genetic testing to prove or disprove paternity needs to be understood in this context. When the very conservative Saudi-based Muslim World League (MWL), for example, took this position, they did so while accepting that genetic fingerprinting is highly reliable and can be used in cases unrelated to family law. The MWL stated that their goal was "protection of people's honor and care for their kinship relations (Clarke 2009, 201)." This response might elicit the question whether a paternity test is a better means of establishing "kinship relations" because it could definitively prove that a child was not the progeny of a woman's husband but in fact was another man's child. Here, their reference to "honor" shows that lineage (*nasab*) is not the only aspect of society which deserves protection. Indeed, when the major "priorities" or "goals" of the law (*maqāṣid al-sharīʿa*) are listed, "honor" is sometimes added as a sixth to the five others: religion, life, property, intellect and lineage. Lineage is a key concept underlying many rules pertaining to sexuality and gender, and will be examined in some detail after we have discussed some of the implications of taking "honor" into consideration in bioethics and family law.

Honor is, no doubt, the least tangible goal, among the other *maqāṣid al-sharīʿa* which deserves protection. Honor in Islamic law is constructed from and protected by a network of laws, procedural rules and manners. The Qur'an assigns a punishment of 80 lashes to those who accuse "chaste women" of unlawful intimacy. Such accusations are deemed lies if there are not four men who swear an oath that they are witnesses — and here jurists elaborated on the Qur'an — to consensual vaginal penetration by a man. Such evidence (unlike proof which could be obtained from a hidden webcam, for example) is exceedingly difficult to obtain. The Qur'an further states that if a man claims to have caught his wife having sex with another man, his only recourse is to swear an oath to the fact; but she can swear an oath to refute his claim. Pre-modern scholars were consistent that the absence of a hymen was not evidence that a woman had had intercourse, and they rejected the legal validity of "virginity tests" which were part of Mediterranean culture (Tucker 1998, 1; 166). Overall, traditional Islamic legal discourse, including *fatwa* literature, shows a concern for attacks on women's sexual morality in particular and puts up many barriers to stop such attacks. Of course, this shows that women were often vulnerable to attacks on their morality and sexual propriety. While defending family or personal "honor" from being degraded by a woman's improper behavior has never been a justification for vigilante justice, also known as "honor killings" in Islamic law, they have been, and still are, a feature of some Muslim cultures. The need to abide by the principle of non-maleficence has thus been raised in places like modern Lebanon where paternity testing has been sought by married men or other family members. A physician specializing in genetic testing in Lebanon told Morgan Clarke (2009, 204), "I stopped doing it because it's a headache in Lebanon — there's no proper recourse after. You don't know what this guy's going to do to his wife and kids."

Privacy is highly valued in traditional Islamic law and ethics. For instance, if a believer has committed a sin, harming only themselves and not another, contrary to the Christian model of confession, he or she should repent only to God and not scandalize the community with stories of his or her sexual transgressions. Likewise, family or friends should not "lift the veil (*sitr*)" that has protected someone from scandal, for this is a divine grace allowing the person an opportunity for repentance and reform. Traditional Islamic law becomes something else altogether when separated from this culture of privacy, limited government intervention and legal pluralism. The calls of modernists and progressives for greater gender equality and freedoms are therefore not just ideological imitations of "the West" but an ethical response to increased state power and technology in modern societies which intrude on privacy and impede a religious ethic of repentance and reformation.[7]

If we consider the value of chastity, for example, we see that in traditional Islamic texts chastity is equally ordained for men as it is for women who have no lawful sexual partner (although men, if they meet the required conditions, are permitted more lawful sexual partners through polygamy and concubinage). In the pre-modern age no reliable birth control was available therefore women always faced a higher risk of having their transgressions discovered if pregnancy resulted. Most Muslims believe that the "protective" religious norms of gender segregation, veiling, and guardianship can be understood in light of this reality. When these protections failed, families might extend the religious principle of compassion and provide "cover" by helping conceal a pregnancy and conducting secret adoptions, despite legal prohibition (Mattson 2005 b, 1–3).

This traditional ethic of privacy: including "covering" another's sins and "don't ask, don't tell" (which applies to all sexual transgressions, including those of the same sex), is increasingly difficult to sustain in contemporary culture. Surveillance technology pervades private and public spaces and it would be difficult in many places to obtain a birth certificate for a child — a necessary document in contemporary life — that would not name the birth mother. While religious scholars continue to resist the use of technology and science to disprove paternity and prove infidelity, the traditional cultural matrix has weakened to the point of breaking in many places. An honest re-evaluation of the ethical priorities related to sexuality and gender seems to be in order. One question which needs to be asked is whether the religious scholars who currently serve as the "experts" in Islamic bioethics are capable of undertaking such a re-evaluation. Ron Shaham, who has studied this issue in Egyptian Islamic courts (and among Orthodox Jews in Israel, whom he sees as close ideological and cultural counterparts), does not believe they can. As in other modern Muslim countries, Egyptian courts have become convinced of the scientific reliability of genetic testing, and DNA evidence is commonly used in criminal proceedings. The majority of religious scholars, however, have absolutely opposed the use of genetic testing in paternity cases. The traditional legal maxim, "The child belongs to the marriage bed" remains here, as elsewhere, the highest legal principle. Shaham (2010, 186) argues that the unassailability of the marital presumption of paternity in Egyptian law "indicates that the social purposes it is designed to serve — defending the integrity of the marital family, protecting against the bastardization of children, and preventing exposure of the immoral conduct of the parents — are still the dominant social norm." Seen from this perspective, it is clearly not "purity" of lineage that is the main concern of the jurists. The more important goals of the law are to keep marriages intact and to keep children within the protective custody of a family. All of this seems, on the balance, positive and beneficial for vulnerable women and children. Shaham (2010, 187–8) argues, nevertheless, that beyond these concerns, the jurists have a greater interest than justice or compassion at stake in these debates and that is their desire to preserve a religious worldview and their authority within that world:

> Traditional elites, especially the religious establishment, fear that the erosion of the marital family without offering an appropriate alternative familial model will bring about undesired social consequences and result in social chaos.... Conflicting worldviews are at play, crucial interests have to be weighed one against the other, and serious questions have to be addressed: Is it in the best interests of a child to have a secured legal paternity or to know who his natural father is? Should the interests of the family as a unit take precedence over the individual interests of the husband who is not the biological father? What are appropriate gender relations? Are out-of-wedlock conjugal relations acceptable? Does an open public debate on sensitive socio-moral issues serve society better than "keeping secrets hidden within houses"?

While some contemporary western societies have embraced "openness" as a value, scientific evidence can not claim that it always does more good than harm.[8] However, sensitive discussions cannot be avoided when the coercive and social restructuring power of the state is involved in regulating sexuality and gender. Where state power and services have increased and centralized, as is the case in contemporary societies, and bioethics regulations are set by the state with the participation of religious scholars, only political openness can bring the perspectives of minorities and marginalized people back into the conversation.

## Shifting Notions of *Nasab* and Its Importance for Discussions about Fertility

In this context, it is important to look more deeply into the way legal scholars invoke the need to protect "lineage." *Nasab* (or *nasl*) is one of the five major "priorities" of the Sacred Law (*maqāṣid al-sharīʿa*), according to the majority of scholars, both traditional and modern. Indeed, modern scholars have tended to elevate the importance of *maqāṣid al-sharīʿa* (the "goals of the sacred law"; henceforth, the *maqāṣid*) as a way to bring a more coherent, holistic, values and outcome-based approach to contemporary legal reasoning.

Abdulaziz Sachedina (2009, 103) describes the place of lineage in the Islamic law: "The preservation of proper lineage (*nasab*) in order for the child to be related to his/her biological parents is one of the main purposes of the sacred law of Islam, the *Sharīʿa*. Accordingly, a child's untainted identity through a legitimate conjugal relationship between a man and a woman in marriage is so essential in Islam and Muslim culture that it is regarded as a child's inalienable right." Sachedina continues, "Under one circumstance, however, Islamic law has refused to grant genealogical recognition to an offspring: when the child is conceived through an act of adultery, an illicit sexual relationship under *Sharīʿa* law." Sachedina (2009, 104) concedes that "in practice, Muslim societies grant lineage to the child's biological parents even if there is no certainty about such an ascription, placing the onus on adult behavior and sparing the child from any future social handicap that might result from the stigma of illegitimacy."

Sachedina's observation is in line with what we have earlier pointed out, that traditional Islamic law and Muslim cultures have aimed to ascribe legitimacy to children, including by allowing for cases of unusually long or short gestation (such as the "sleeping child"). Yet, in discussing the denial of the validity of procedures such as sperm or egg donation and gestational surrogacy, which is the majority *Sunni* position

(Al-Bar and Chamsi-Pasha 2015, 175–8), Sachedina often resorts to a notion of purity/impurity in lineage, using words such as "unblemished," "taint," and "sully." I am deeply concerned that this terminology only contributes to the stigmatization of some children who, after all, are not responsible for the manner of their conception. In this regard it is important to remember that the majority of scholars have asserted that the human body is substantially pure; in the words of Imam al-Shafiʿī: "no one who is alive from the children of Adam is substantially impure (Katz 2002, 167; Al-Shafiʿī 1989, 1; 104)."

Perhaps we need to step back and ask whether the major rationale for making *nasab* a priority in the law is the protection of children, or the protection of "pure" bloodlines? It seems that the two goals are so intertwined in the law, that for many, they cannot be separated. If the blood relationship between parent and child is so important, and it is increasingly difficult in modern society to "cover" an unlawful pregnancy, scholars might reconsider the use of paternity testing to assign lineage to a child born out of marriage. After all, in traditional Islamic law marriage is the only licit sexual relationship. Before the abolition of slavery, the child of a concubine was given all the same rights of lineage and support as a child born of marriage. What is notable in this regard is that these rights were instituted by the early caliph ʿUmar ibn al-Khaṭṭāb out of compassion for a child and his mother. When he was criticized by some men for burdening them with more responsibilities in this regard, ʿUmar cited the Qurʾanic value of "doing good" (*al-maʿrūf*) as justification for making this law (Mattson 1999, 126; 150).

Jasser Auda (2008, 23–4) notes that most modern scholars have developed *nasab* into "a family-oriented theory." The influential Tunisian jurist Ibn ʿAshūr, for example, made "care for the family" a goal in its own right. It is not only modernist scholars, but some traditionalists too who have substituted "family" or "children" for "paternity" or "lineage" as the meaning of *nasab*. Contemporary American *Mālikī* scholar Umar Faruq Abd-Allah (2007, 19) identifies the "preservation of children" as the priority. This, he says, "focuses on children but entails everything essential to the welfare of the family. It takes in marriage, parenting, caring for the disabled, and so forth. It necessitates guarding against social evils like the abuse of children, spouses, and the elderly."

Here it becomes evident that elevating the *maqāṣid* in modern Islamic legal discourse, while perhaps providing broad, unifying values to frame discussions about religion and family life, nevertheless leaves us with no consensus about how the priorities should be defined and ranked. We see vastly different views among Muslims on whether the main priority is to protect children, to produce children, or to provide a lawful outlet for sexual activity, even if there is no intention to produce children. For example, religious scholars who previously took the position that birth control is prohibited have moved in recent decades to recommending it as a means of having healthier, better cared-for children (Bennett 2005, 115; Rispler-Haim 1993, 12–4). This outcome is certainly welcomed by men and women. Using birth control can, however, have multiple and diverse impacts on men, women, and their relationships. Scholars have always maintained that birth control cannot be used within a marriage without the consent of both partners. The impact of pre-modern versus modern forms of birth control, however, is tremendously different. Pre-modern birth control was not as safe and certainly not nearly as reliable as modern methods, so couples engaging in sexual relations were normally taking a significant risk that this would result in a pregnancy. In contrast, it is now possible to prevent conception completely so that one can engage in a sexual relationship without there being any chance of forming of a family. Perhaps this explains the apparent increase in multiple serial, secret and *de facto* temporary marriages, a development which many see as often exploitative of women (Fadel 2016; Kaukab 2016). On the other hand, spacing or limiting the number of pregnancies can save women's lives and allow them more time and resources to develop and employ capacities other than reproductive and parental. In some cases, there can be a shift in the identities of the husband and wife from being primarily parents, to being a couple where intimacy and friendship are paramount. The social consequences completely severing reproduction from sexual relations have not been well-studied among contemporary Muslims remains an open question whether intimacy and friendship strengthen, or weaken the concept of "family."

Some continue to see the proliferation of children as an absolute benefit, as long as a man has the means to financially support these children. Where having numerous children is seen as the primary purpose of marriage and a religious, or religiously sanctioned cultural value, a Muslim man has traditionally been encouraged to engage in polygamy if his wife is infertile or to simply father as many children as he can afford (Doi 1984, 144–54). In this context, the development of modern fertility treatments has been welcomed as a "marriage savior" by many Muslims subject to this kind of religiously sanctioned cultural pressure to reproduce. There appears to be universal acceptance of *in vitro* fertilisation as long as the egg and sperm are from a married couple and the embryo is implanted in the womb of the wife. There is an increasing demand among Muslims, however, to expand the range of permissible fertility treatments and reproductive technologies in order to save marriages. In *Shi'ite* jurisprudence in particular, which allows more innovation in legal reasoning (*ijtihād*), scholars increasingly seem willing to prioritize stabilizing a married couple's relationship above ensuring purity of lineage. Ayatollah Khamenei was a groundbreaker in this regard, permitting the use of donated gametes as long as illicit sexual contact is not involved (Clarke 2009, 191–2; Inhorn 2006, 350–1). Other scholars and most Muslims did not embrace this view in large numbers; however, this may be changing. Iran, for example, is reporting significant decreases in fertility, which is attributed (rightly or wrongly) to environmental pollution. A huge increase in demand for reproductive assistance is nudging Iranian society in the direction of accepting more assited reproductive procedures, including the use of donated embryos which can be considered to have "their own identity" and thus can be implanted in a woman's body, unlike non-spousal sperm (*Iranians Fighting Rising Infertility* 2015).

One wonders if it is not time to put more emphasis on the protection of existing children in Islamic bioethics over the concern for purity of lineage and the proliferation of children. Of course, if couples insist on dedicating personal financial resources to lawful fertility treatments, that is their right. But in the interest of justice — a key Qur'anic value, as well as a major concern of bioethics — shelter, security, nutrition, healthcare, and education for orphaned, abandoned, and impoverished children should be given greater priority in public budgets. Textbooks on Islamic bioethics consistently marginalize adoption and fostering, although the Prophet Muhammad could not have been more adamant about the importance of caring for needy children. To say that "adoption is prohibited" is misleading, given that open adoptions, which are functionally equivalent to Islamic fostering, are common in society today (Mattson 2005b, 1). The medical intervention relevant in this regard is lactation stimulation which many women seek to create the legal bond of "milk-mother" with the fostered child. More research could also be done on the way attachment can be stimulated in men who foster children, so they feel closeness with the child and thus feel less compelled to seek expensive and risky fertility treatments.

## Sexuality and Gender Identity

For those interested in a liberal Islam which allows individuals to live according to their own understanding of the religion, the methods and authority of traditional Islamic scholars and their claims that their "consensus (*ijma'*)" on matters is the law will be directly challenged. The priorities and ethics of a progressive methodology regarding sexuality are described here, for example, by Scott Kugle (2010):

> The reformist or progressive approach must take into account new possibilities for human fulfillment in increasingly non-patriarchal societies like those evolving under democratic institutions, where Muslims are living as minority communities and fellow citizens. In these new environments, it is possible for homosexual relationships to be based on ethical reciprocity, trust, justice, and love, just as heterosexual relationships ought to be based on these values in the ethical vision of the Qur'an. What matters is not the sex of the partner with whom one forms a partnership, as long as that partnership is contractual on par with legal custom. Rather, what matters is the ethical nature of the relationship one has within the constraints of one's internal disposition, which includes sexual orientation and gender identity.

Establishing "ethical reciprocity" as a legitimate basis for Islamic marriage would allow non-traditional marriages including same-sex marriages, if same-sex intimacy is not deemed immoral. The majority of Muslims, it seems, remain unconvinced by revisionist readings of the Qur'an in this direction. At the same time, there is a great deal of evidence that pre-modern Muslims treated same-sex attraction as commonplace (El-Rouayheb 2005; Gessinger 2011, 28–35). Since there is no legal mechanism to legitimize same-sex intimacy in traditional Islamic law, however, it was recommended to suppress such desires with ascetic practices such as fasting and avoiding situations of temptation. The pre-modern culture of privacy we have already discussed has been widely understood to have facilitated discrete, perhaps even life-long, same-sex partnerships within Muslim societies.

Most Islamic bioethics textbooks give little attention to sexuality of any kind, thus neglecting many serious issues related to psychological, physical, and public health. Often scholars seem to feel that harmful behavior is best prevented by asserting the rules of lawful sexual intimacy. There is little evidence that most religious scholars are interested in pursuing harm reduction policies, even though certainly some Muslims engage in risky sexual behaviors which may result, among other harms, in the spread of sexually transmitted diseases. Even where there is evidence that large numbers of unmarried Muslim youth are engaged in unprotected sexual contact, religious scholars and communities often are opposed to public sex education programs (Ahmed *et al.* 2015). This is not necessarily an irrational response to the situation when many families believe they can best teach their own children. The reality is, however, that not all parents will do a good job empowering children with the knowledge and resources they need to protect themselves.

Research done among American Muslims shows that many do not learn about sex from parents or school; instead, they acquire misinformation from peers and seek out pornography on the internet. The result is that some youth are vulnerable to sexual abuse and violence, and have problems with intimacy in their marriages (Mohajir 2016). The ethical principle that there is a communal responsibility (*fard kifayah*) to protect all children and to nurture their capacities is relevant in this context. If the Muslim community has a faith-based objection to the de-stigmatization of extra-marital sexual contact in public education, then it is their responsibility to provide appropriate sex education which gives children the knowledge and resources they need to protect themselves from predators, diseases, and other harms.

It is also important that women, as well as men, are given accurate information about sexual desire and enjoyment. Traditional and modern religious texts need to be scrutinized because they run the gamut in this regard; one can find discourses emphasizing women's rights and needs and others which are demeaning to women.[9] Broad statements are sometimes made about the difference between men's and women's sexual needs and desires on the basis of Galenic theories of "active" masculinity and "passive" or "receptive" femininity (Avicenna 1970, 100; Murata 1992, 196; Winter 2011). The 14th century text by Ibn Qayyim al-Jawziyya on the so-called "Prophetic medicine" finds wide circulation in the original Arabic and in translation among contemporary Muslims who often naively accept the contents as religiously normative. Many of the teachings in this text and in this genre in general are probably benign or beneficial. Some of the statements, however, reinforce harmful paradigms of male superiority and can have a negative impact on women's and men's self-esteem and enjoyment of sex. For example, Ibn Qayyim (1998, 185) says, "the worst (sexual) position is for the woman to be on top, and that he has intercourse with her lying on his back. For this is contrary to the natural form in which God made the man and woman, or rather the species of male and female … the woman is passive both by nature and by law. If she should be the active partner, she contravenes the demands of nature and the law." Many traditional scholars viewed strong sexual desire in women so problematic, that it necessitated genital cutting (FGC). Overwhelming scientific evidence of the harmful effects of FGC, in addition to sustained advocacy by women's rights organizations, has brought many scholars in recent times to the conclusion that FGC is religiously prohibited mutilation, etc. (Rispler-Haim 1993, 85–90; Kassamali 2006, 132). The increasing acceptance of this position should be seen as a victory for Islamic bioethics, whereby the principles of non-maleficence and justice have triumphed over bad science, patriarchy, and injustice.

Turning our attention to another, somewhat related concern, gender identity is a topic that has been addressed relatively openly by traditional Islamic scholars due to the appearance in *hadith* literature of the *mukhannath,* a term that is variously translated as "effeminacy, transvestism, transsexualism, or hermaphroditism." Lagrange (2003, 421) says this "puzzling inconsistency" can be understood "when one considers that the term refers to various failings to achieve masculinity in its behavioral features." In traditional Muslim societies, nevertheless, there seems to have always been a distinctive cultural and even religious role for this non-masculine male (Scalenghe 2014, 124–62; Wikan 1982). The recent development of gender-reassignment surgeries and hormone therapies are allowing and, in some cases, pushing such people to choose one of two gender binaries (Rispler-Haim 1993, 49). In Iran where gender reassignment surgery is allowed, concerns have been raised that non-transgender gay people are essentially being coerced into surgery because there is no other lawful means for them to marry (Jafari 2014). As for hermaphroditism, the question arises whether Islamic bioethics can view this as part of God-created human diversity, or whether it is a medical condition which should be treated in order to ensure that all people fit into a binary gender system of classification. Sachedina (2009, 192–3) seems convinced that cultural norms in Muslims societies, as well as traditional jurisprudence, demand binary gender identity and this is why there is widespread support among Muslim scholars for surgical solutions to achieve this goal. No doubt we will see increasing advocacy in the opposite direction by those who deny that sex designation as male or female is "critical for an individual's interaction and relationships with others in society."

## Conclusion

It is my perspective that it is not always necessary to adopt a radically non-traditional legal hermeneutic to bring about significant changes in the law. Where Islamic legal authority is less hierarchical, state-enforced, and patriarchal, new perspectives can be put forward, debated, and eventually integrated into the range of acceptable positions within a framework of legal pluralism. Asserting that this is the intellectual context within which we are surveying Islamic bioethics in this collection, I suggest that reasonable arguments can be made for alternative priorities and solutions for a number of issues related to sexuality and gender in Islamic bioethics. Evidence-based science is critical in Islamic bioethics, but it is important to avoid "scientism," a tendency in much of modern Islamic discourse (Iqbal 2015, 1691). Neither should Islamic bioethics be reduced to legalism. The Islamic values of compassion; helping the weak; restoration of family and community ties; and prioritizing a believer's relationship with God always need to be recognized. Finally, the Islamic requirement of "consultation (*shura*)" must be fullfiled in any community decisions, and this means that more effort needs to be made to include women and non-gender conforming Muslims in discussions of Islamic bioethics.

## Notes

1   Hallaq notes that "the traditional competence of the ruler's *siyāsa sharʿiyya* has been expended beyond recognition." Hallaq, W. 2009. *Sharīʿa: Theory, Practice, Transformations.* Cambridge, UK: Cambridge University Press, 448.

2   The clash between Ahmad ibn Hanbal and the Abbasid scholars in 9th century Baghdad is a famous example; see: Mattson, I. 2013. *The Story of the Qurʾan: Its History and Place in Muslim Life.* Rev. 2nd ed. Malden, MA: Wiley-Blackwell, 144–5.

3   Notable in this regard is the work of Mohammad Akram Nadwi summarized in his book: Nadwi, M. A. 2007. *Al-Muhaddithat: the Women Scholars in Islam.* Oxford: Interface Publications.

4   See, for example, the collection of essays dedicated to feminist critiques of traditional assertions of male guardianship: Mir-Hosseini, Z., Al-Sharmani, M. and Rumminger, J. (eds.). 2015. *Men in Charge? Rethinking Authority in Muslim Legal Tradition.* London: Oneworld.

5   One wonders if the authors even understand well the actual role of women in the society in which they work, given that contemporary Saudi women have attained significant levels of wealth, educational achievement, and business success. See, for example, Raval, A. 2015. Saudi Women Take the Business Path. *Financial Times,* December 22, 2015. Available at: http://www.ft.com/cms/s/0/a4d20e58-8a33-11e5-90de-f44762bf9896.html#axzz4IqoDCDJf.

6   "Some of the results of effective Islamic spiritual care are an increase in hope, which acknowledges the fact that Allah is omnipotent and omnipresent and is the ultimate recourse. Such care gives hope and strength to the distressed soul, eliminates or reduces despair and brings the supplicant closer to the Creator, strengthening the bond between them, and returns the client to the community." Isgandarova, N. 2011. *Effective Islamic Spiritual Care: Foundations and Practices of Imams and Other Muslim Spiritual Caregivers.* Wilfred Laurier University Doctor of Ministry Thesis, 86.

7   Mohammad Hashim Kamali is a strong proponent of this view in his works such as: Kamali, M. H. 2008. *The Right to Life, Security, Privacy and Ownership in Islam.* Cambridge, UK: The Islamic Texts Society.

8   For example, there is some evidence that greater openness about suicide in order to remove stigma might lead to more suicides. Bielski, Z. 2010. A Teen's

Suicide Rekindles Debate over Openness. *The Globe and Mail,* November 18, 2010. Availableat:http://www.theglobeandmail.com/life/health-and-fitness/health/conditions/a-teens-suicide-rekindles-debate-over-openness/article 595321/.

9   Such as those extensively documented and refuted by Khaled Abou El Fadl in his work: Fadl, K. A. E. 2001. *Speaking in God's Name: Islamic Law, Authority and Women.* Oxford: Oneworld, 209–62.

## References

Abd-Allah, U. F. 2007. *Living Islam with Purpose.* Chicago: Nawawi Foundation.

Ahmed, S., Patel, S. and Hashem, H. 2015. *State of American Muslim Youth: Research and Recommendations.* [n.p.] (USA): The Family and Youth Institute and Institute for Social Policy Understanding.

al-Jawziyya, Ibn Qayyim. 1998. *Medicine of the Prophet.* Trans. Johnstone, P. Cambridge, UK: The Islamic Texts Society.

Ali, K. 2016. *Sexual Ethics and Islam: Feminist Reflections on Qur'an, Hadith, and Jurisprudence.* 2nd ed. Oxford: Oneworld.

Ansari, Z. 2015. Blurred Lines: Women, "Celebrity" Shaykhs, and Spiritual Abuse. Available at: http://muslimmatters.org/2015/05/27/blurred-lines-women-celebrity-shaykhs-spiritual-abuse/.

Al-Shafiʻi, M. ibn I. 1989. *Al-Umm,* 8 vols. Cairo: Dar al-Ghada al-ʻArabi.

Auda, J. 2008. *Maqāṣid Al-Sharīʻah: A Beginner's Guide.* Occasional papers series 14. London and Washington: The International Institute of Islamic Thought.

Avicenna. 1970. *A Treatise on the Canon of Medicine of Avicenna, Incorporating a Translation of the First Book.* Trans. Gruner O. C. Reprint of 1930 Luzac publication. New York: Augustus M. Kelley.

Al-Bar, M. A. and Chamsi-Pasha, H. 2015. *Contemporary Bioethics: Islamic Perspective.* Heidelberg, etc: Springer Open.

Bennett, L. R. 2005. *Women, Islam and Modernity: Single Women, Sexuality, and Reproductive Health in Contemporary Indonesia.* London: Routledge Curzon.

Bin Bayyah, A. *Ruling on Marriage Intended for Securing some Benefit.* Available at: http://binbayyah.net/english/2012/01/28/ruling-on-marriage-intended-for-securing-some-benefit/.

Bowen, D. L. 2006. Reproduction: Abortion and Islam — Overview. In: Joseph, S. (ed.). *Encyclopedia of Women and Islamic Cultures, Volume III: Family, Body, Sexuality and Health.* Leiden and Boston: Brill.

Caldwell, B. 2006. Reproduction: Infertility — South Asia. In: Joseph, S. (ed.). *Encyclopedia of Women and Islamic Cultures, Volume III: Family, Body, Sexuality and Health.* Leiden and Boston: Brill.

Clarke, M. 2009. *Islam and New Kinship: Reproductive Technology and the Shariah in Lebanon.* New York and Oxford: Berghahn Books.

El Shakry, O. 2006. Science: Medicalization and the Female Body — Overview. In: Joseph, S. (ed.). *Encyclopedia of Women and Islamic Cultures, Volume III: Family, Body, Sexuality and Health.* Leiden and Boston: Brill.

El-Rouayheb, K. 2005. *Before Homosexuality in the Arab-Islamic World, 1500-1800.* Chicago: University of Chicago Press.

Fadel, M. 2016. *Not All Marriages Are Equal: Islamic Marriage, Temporary Marriage, Secret Marriage and Polygamous Marriage.* Available from: http://www.altmuslimah.com/2016/03/not-marriages-equal-islamic-marriage-temporary-marriage-secret-marriage-polygamous-marriage/.

Gessinger, A. 2011. Islam and Same-Sex Sexuality in History: Cultural and Religious Perspectives. In: *Muslim LGBT Inclusion Project — Final Report.* New York: Intersections International.

Inhorn, M. C. Reproduction: New Technologies — Overview. In: Joseph, S. (ed.). *Encyclopedia of Women and Islamic Cultures, Volume III: Family, Body, Sexuality and Health.* Leiden and Boston: Brill.

Iqbal, M. 2015. Scientific Commentary on the Qur'an. In: Nasr, S. H., Dahli, et al. *The Study Qur'an: A New Translation and Commentary.* New York: HarperCollins, 1679–93.

Iranians Fight Rising Infertility and Taboos. 2015. *Almonitor,* August 16. Available at: http://www.al-monitor.com/pulse/afp/2016/08/iran-health-children-religion.html.

Jafari, F. 2014. Transsexuality Under Surveillance in Iran: Clerical Control of Khomeini's Fatwas. *Journal of Middle East Women's Studies,* 10(2), 31–51.

Jansen, W. 2000. Sleeping in the Womb: Protracted Pregnancies in the Maghreb. *The Muslim World* 90(1/2), 218–37.

Kassamali, N. 2006. Genital Cutting: Africa and the Middle East. In: Joseph, S. (ed.). *Encyclopedia of Women and Islamic Cultures, Volume III: Family, Body, Sexuality and Health.* Leiden and Boston: Brill.

Katz, M. H. 2002. *Body of Text: The Emergence of the Sunnī Law of Ritual Purity.* Albany: State University of New York Press.

Kaukab, S. 2016. Secret Marriages, Spiritual Abuse, and Our Scholars: An Introduction to 'Not All Marriages are Equal'. *Almuslimah*, March 13. Available at: http://www.altmuslimah.com/2016/03/secret-marriages-morality-scholars-introduction-not-marriages-equal-2/.

Kugle, S. S. al-H. 2010. *Homosexuality in Islam: Critical Reflections on Gay, Lesbian, and Transgender Muslims*. Oxford: Oneworld.

Lagrange, F. 2003. Sexualities and Queer Studies. In: Joseph, S. (ed.). *Encyclopedia of Women and Islamic Cultures, Volume I: Methodologies, Paradigms and Sources*. Leiden; Boston: Brill.

Mattson, I. 1999. *A Believing Slave is Better Than an Unbeliever: Status and Community in Early Islamic Society and Law*. University of Chicago doctoral dissertation.

Mattson, I. 2005a. Women, Gender and Family Law: Early Period 7th–late 18th centuries. In: Joseph, S. (ed.). *Encyclopedia of Women and Islamic Cultures, Volume II: Family, Law and Politics*. Leiden and Boston: Brill.

Mattson, I. 2005b. Adoption and Fosterage. In: Joseph, S. (ed.). *Encyclopedia of Women and Islamic Cultures, Volume II: Family, Law and Politics*. Leiden and Boston: Brill.

Mohajir, N. 2016. *Starting the Conversation*. [n.p.]: Heart Women and Girls. Available at: http://heartwomenandgirls.org/publications/.

Murata, S. 1992. *The Tao of Islam: A Sourcebook on Gender Relationships in Islamic Thought*. Albany, NY: State University of New York Press.

Quraishi, A. 2010. What is Sharia and Is It Creepy? *The Islamic Monthly*, Winter/Spring, 25. Available at: http://theislamicmonthly.com/what-is-sharia-and-is-it-creepy/.

Rauf, F. 2015. *Defining Islamic Statehood: Measuring and Indexing Contemporary Muslim States*. Basingstoke, UK: Palgrave Macmillan.

Rispler-Chaim, V. 1993. *Islamic Medical Ethics in the Twentieth Century*. Leiden: Brill.

Sachedina, A. 2009. *Islamic Biomedical Ethics*. New York: Oxford University Press.

Scalenghe, S. 2014. *Disability in the Ottoman Arab World, 1500–1800*. Cambridge: Cambridge University Press.

Semerdjian, E. 2008. *Off the Straight Path: Illicit Sex, Law and Community in Ottoman Aleppo*. Syracuse: Syracuse University Press.

Shaham, R. 2010. *The Expert Witness in Islamic Courts: Medicine and Crafts in the Service of the Law*. Chicago: The University of Chicago Press.

Shahidan, H. 2008. Contesting Discourses of Sexuality in Post-Revolutionary Iran. In: İlkkaracan, P. (ed.). *Deconstructing Sexuality in the Middle East: Challenges and Discourses*. Aldershot: Ashgate.

Shaikh, S. 2015. Islamic Law, Sufism and Gender: Rethinking the Terms of the Debate. In: Mir-Hosseini, Z., Al-Sharmani, M. and Rumminger, J. (ed.). *Men in Charge? Rethinking Authority in Muslim Legal Tradition*. London: Oneworld.

Stimler, M. S. 2006. Reproduction: Medicalization of — Arab States. In: Joseph, S. (ed.). *Encyclopedia of Women and Islamic Cultures, Volume III, Family, Body, Sexuality and Health*. Leiden: Brill.

Tucker, J. E. 1998. *In the House of the Law: Gender and Islamic Law in Ottoman Syria and Palestine*. Berkeley: University of California Press.

Wadud, A. 2006. *Inside the Gender Jihad: Women's Reform in Islam*. Oxford, UK: Oneworld.

Weiss, B. 1998. *The Spirit of Islamic Law*. Athens, GA: University of Georgia Press.

Wikan, U. 1982. *Behind the Veil in Arabia: Women in Oman*. Chicago: University of Chicago.

Winter, T. J. 2011. *The Human Person in Islam*. Paper presented at the 2nd Muslim–Catholic Forum, Baptism Site, Jordan, November 21–23, 2011. Amman: The Royal Aal al-Bayt Institute for Islamic Thought.

# CHAPTER FIVE

## The Physician–Patient Relationship
## in an Islamic Context

### *Mohammad Ali Albar and Hassan Chamsi-Pasha*

### Summary

The physician–patient relationship constitutes one of the foundations of contemporary medical ethics. It is the cornerstone of the practice of medicine and essential for delivering high-quality healthcare. In the current era, financial targets, sophisticated diagnostics, media, and widespread access to the internet, all distract from the central, human interaction between a physician and patient. This chapter reviews some of the critical elements in a trusting relationship, such as obtaining informed consent; protecting confidentiality; respecting cultural norms and modesty; and breaking bad news. To establish a good therapeutic relationship, the physician's communication skills are very critical and aid in developing a culturally sensitive understanding of the patient's values and wishes. Formal training to develop communication skills and in breaking bad news is strongly encouraged.

## Introduction

The physician–patient relationship (PPR) is a central concern of both medical ethics and practice, as it stresses how the interaction between the doctor and patient ought to be. The relationship begins with the first

85

consultation. Hence it is very important to conduct this first visit in a proper and receptive manner. Consulting with a patient is a complicated skill that is gradually learned during medical training and is more effectively undertaken as the physician gains experience (Terpstra 2012). Beyond the consulting rooms, for instance in the hospital ward, the simple dyadic PPR is far more complex as it involves many other people including the patient's family and neighbors, as well other team members, such as nurses, therapists, and pharmacists (Balint 2008).

It has been proposed that an ideal PPR has six components, namely voluntary choice, physician's competence, good communication, continuity of care, physician's empathy, and absence of conflict of interest. A poor PPR, on the other hand, has been proven to be a major hurdle for both physicians and patients to overcome, and will eventually affect the quality of healthcare provided as well as the ability of the patients to cope with their illness. In the case of poor PPR, patients may not comply with the doctor's advice; they may practice doctor-shopping by frequently changing their physicians; may remain anxious; may choose fraudulent or other non-scientific forms of treatment; and may experience a significant increase in medical expenses (Terpstra 2012).

The nature of the PPR has changed dramatically over the years, mostly due to the commercialization and privatization of health sector services. Physicians sometimes, ask for unnecessary medical tests or may give over-prescriptions, just to be safe or to avoid litigation. There is also a remarkable decline in human touch or empathy; and a significant rise in unhealthy competition among physicians.

Modern medical science is increasingly technology-based with substantial investment behind the technology. Patients, therefore, may think physicians have a financial interest in using the technology. Poor patients may also see a bleak financial future when considering the costly medicine and expensive investigations. He looks blankly at the prescription as if he sees the paper documenting the sale of his last belongings (Islam 2012).

Several factors, such as socio-cultural determinants, poor communication skills, use of medical terminology by the clinicians, not listening to the patient's complaints, and difference between the physician's objectives and the patient's expectations, have together created a wide gap in the relationship between physicians and their patients. All these factors have caused a massive impact on the trust level and the bonding pattern between physicians and their patients (Banerjee 2012). Physicians must understand their patients' distress cordially and to treat the patient's disease and not just the symptoms. Without full understanding of the cultural background of the patient, it is impossible to establish an effective and trusting relationship with the patient.

## The Physician's Responsibilities in Islam

It is incumbent of Muslim community to train health professionals, and it is considered a sin for the whole community if it does not train the required number of healthcare professionals. Preservation of life entails seeking a remedy, and that requires the knowledge of medicine. Imam Shafi'i (d. 820/204 AH) said that knowledge (science) has two main branches: one of religion and the second of human body (medicine) (*al ilm ilman, ilm al adyan* and *ilm al abdan*).

Al Izz ibn Abdul Salam, a renowned Islamic jurist (d. 1243/660 AH) in his book *Qawa'id al Ahkam* (*Basics of Rulings*), said: "The aim of medicine, like the aim of Islamic law (*Shari'a*), is to procure the utility or benefit (*maslaha*) of human beings, bringing safety and health to them and warding off the harm of injuries and ailments, as much as possible." He also said: "The aim of medicine is to preserve health; restore it when it is lost; remove ailment or reduce its effects".

However, to reach that goal it may be essential to accept the lesser harm, in order to ward off a greater one; or lose a certain benefit to procure a greater one. This is a very pragmatic attitude, which is widely accepted, in Islamic jurisprudence, and it is frequently applied in daily practice in all fields including medicine (Albar and Chamsi-Pasha 2015).

The Qur'an and sayings of the Prophet of Islam established the morality and mode of conduct of physicians and surgeons. The Prophet gave many rules regarding seeking remedy, and the importance of consent. Islamic jurists require the physicians to be competent and obtain a license to practice medicine. He also should get the consent of the patient or his guardian if the patient is not competent, otherwise he would be liable (*zamen*).

The Qur'an and *Sunna* teach the Muslim physicians the importance of possessing good manners (*khuluq*) which incorporate mercy, patience, tolerance, kindness, and honesty, while avoiding selfishness, arrogance, and anger (Arawi 2011).

Importantly, there is also great emphasis placed on acting beneficently. The term beneficence implies acts of mercy, kindness, charity, altruism, love, and humanity. Beneficence is intimate with the principle of non-maleficence, but it is so dominant to other ethical principles that it can be claimed that the principles of beneficence and non-maleficence are the starting point in all kinds of human relations. This is perhaps an interesting point when compared to the application of medical ethics in western countries where beneficence and non-maleficence are not necessarily the starting point. In certain cases the principle of individual autonomy is often considered more important and can outweigh other ethical principles (such as the case of euthanasia, which is now increasing practiced in western European countries).

The Qur'an and *hadiths* of the Prophet Muhammad are full of verses (*ayat*) and sayings of the Prophet enjoining persons to do good and refrain from doing harm (Chamsi-Pasha and Albar 2013a). The Qur'an says: "Whoever has done an atom's weight of good will see it. And whoever has done an atom's weight of evil will see it" (99: 7-8).

One of the earliest and most thorough books on medical ethics is entitled *Practical Ethics of the Physician* (*Adab al-Tabib*) by Ishaq ibn Ali al-Ruhawi. Al-Ruhawi was a contemporary of Abu Bakr Al-Razi (Rhazes) and lived in the second-half of the 9th century AD. This book was translated into English by Martin Levey in 1967. Al-Ruhawi stated that the true physician is the one who fears God; the word fear here includes love and respect. His conscience is his censor, and he is aware that God's eye is ever watching. Rhazes had also written a book fully devoted to medical ethics called *Medical Ethics* (*Akhlaq al-Tabib*). To establish such opinions in a well-organized book over a thousand years ago is quite significant. These ideas still maintain their relevance nowadays and are laid down in several ethical codes of medicine (Chamsi-Pasha and Albar 2013b).

According to Rhazes, the physician has duties to patients. The first of which is to treat the patients kindly, not to be rude or aggressive but soft-spoken, compassionate, and behave modestly. Rhazes stresses that the second duty is to keep the secrets they have learnt during the treatment process of their patients. This principle of confidentiality, put forward by Rhazes, is embodied in the Hippocratic Oath. Another duty is to encourage the patient psychologically. The physician should encourage patients, even those who have no hope of recovering from their diseases, and instill some hope in them. He should also stress the virtue of patience (*sabr*). To Rhazes, another duty of the physician to his patients is to treat the patients equally regardless of their wealth or social status. The aim of the physician should not be the money he will get after treatment but the cure. Physicians should be even more eager to cure the poor and homeless than curing the rich. On the other hand, the patient has also duties to the physician. According to Rhazes, the first thing for a patient to fulfill is to treat the physician kindly and to talk gently. Rhazes, on this point, supports Hippocrates by quoting his words. "Find your physician and prepare him before you need him" (Rhazes 2001).

Patients and students of medicine frequently complain about attending physicians who do not want to spend more than minimal time with them and lack patience in responding to worries or queries. The physicians should always be honest, benefit their patients, and speak kind words to others. The *Sunna* warns against selfishness and arrogance, two major transgressions that have marked modern medicine. Several studies revealed the public dismay at the attitudes of physicians who often act with superiority towards their colleagues and patients. A primary complaint commonly found in these studies is that physicians are often arrogant and prideful. The Prophet of Islam said: "Allah will not look, on the Day of Resurrection, at a person who drags his garment (*izār*) (behind him) out of pride and arrogance (Sahīh Al-Bukhārī 2002).

The physician must behave in a way that does not abuse the societal advantage given to him or her directly or indirectly. With the advancement of diagnostic medical technology, many modern physicians refer their patients for sophisticated investigations without even performing a physical examination, thus failing to treat the patient as a human and instead treating the patient as a medical case, number, or a disease to be dealt with as quickly as possible. With health systems facing financial problems, medicine is turning into a market place and physicians often see their patients as customers. Although, in private practice, the doctor's fees are his lawful right and his earnings are legitimate, many medical codes of ethics request that physicians waive their fees for poor patients. In reality, waivers are often granted to rich and influential patients who could provide physicians with societal benefits (Arawi 2011). In Islam, the Prophet has advised to "feed the hungry, visit the sick and set free the captives" (Saḥīḥ Al-Bukhārī 2002).

The medical profession is unique in that the patient should not be denied the service even if he cannot afford the fee. In the case of a needy person suffering from a medical necessity or emergency, it is the doctor's duty to be considerate and kind, and avoid charging fees which would add a further burden atop of the ailment. According to Islamic teaching, for as you give to the poor, it is to God you are giving and alms-giving is not only due on material possessions but also on knowledge and skills. Fully entitled to make a decent living and earn a legitimate income, a physician shall always honor the high standards of his profession and hold it in the highest regard; never prescribing to activities of propaganda, receiving a commission, or cutting earnings or similar wrongdoings. The way a physician deals with his various patients is a perfect portrayal of his personal and professional integrity. The sphere of a physician's charity, nicety, patience, and tolerance should be large enough to encompass the patient's relatives, friends and those who care for or worry about the patient, but without compromising the dictates of "Professional secrecy" (Islamic Code of Medical Ethics 1981). It is imperative for a Muslim physician to always remember the Prophet Muhammad saying: "The best among you are those who have the best manner and character (Saḥīḥ Al-Bukhārī 2002).

## The Role of Family in Islamic Societies

One major factor that must be considered in the care of Muslim patients is the importance of the family. The fundamental roles of education, spiritual development, and distribution of traditions and practices are shared within the context of a stable family. This unit provides both security and support for its members and often includes close relatives. Elders are treated with kindness and respect, and children are loved and cherished (Ott 2003). Even in the context of a hospitalization, parents often assume direct responsibility for the care of their children.

It is not uncommon for elderly parents to care for their sick adult children, or for their distant relatives. At the time of hospitalization, one or both parents request to remain with the child at all times. Similarly, adult children are obliged to care for their parents, and this responsibility frequently extends to both in-laws and grandchildren. However, this might be different from the western cultures. Allowing relatives to remain with their family member after visiting hours, and providing additional bedding and meals to relatives, so their vigil is more comfortable, permits parents or children to fulfill their family obligation. Likewise, permitting a parent or family member to attend simple procedures or to accompany his or her loved one to surgery would be beneficial. However this may be prohibited if the relative is prone to fainting when seeing blood or operative interventions, or if the relative may interfere during the operation. During such events, relatives often recite prayers or read the Qur'an, appealing for the cure of their loved ones. Recognizing family obligations and appreciating their importance is a key step in caring for Muslim families (Hussain 2010). Moreover, visiting family and friends in the hospital is extremely important in Islam. Muslims are required to visit those who are sick or injured and provide patients and their families with comfort and support. The Prophet says: "A Muslim visiting his sick Muslim brother will continue to be in the harvest of paradise until he or she returns home" (Sahih Muslim). The teachings of Islam recommend Muslims not only meet with those who are ill but also converse with them, provide words of encouragement, and pray for their well-being and prompt recovery. This important obligation is vital to the care of Muslim patients, and measures should be taken to accommodate these visitations (Hussain 2010; Ott 2003). However, it is important to recognize that visitations may impose additional stress on the nursing staff or adjacent patients sharing semi-private rooms. This concern is supported by a recent survey of nursing staff caring for Muslim patients in an intensive-care unit in Saudi Arabia showing that families and friends cause additional demands and distractions to the nursing staff (Halligan 2006).

## Communication and Informed Consent

One of the most important roles of physicians is to facilitate communication with their patients. Providing information to patients for their full understanding of the possible treatment options and appreciation of each option's risks and benefits is vital to the success of a therapeutic relationship between physicians and their patients. Many barriers to communication can arise when Muslim patients are treated in the clinic or hospital. Regardless of the means, overcoming language barriers is mandatory for effective communication. Physicians should talk with patients about future issues that will affect their health and also with other team members about the patients they care together (Frey 2013). Basic requirements of informed consent include a discussion and an enumeration of risks, benefits, as well as presenting the alternatives if they exist. This discussion should address serious as well as common risks. Patients should be encouraged to ask question and express their concerns and the process should be voluntary and without coercion. In addition, this procedure must be witnessed (Packer 2011).

The discussion must be understood by all parties involved. An interpreter may be beneficial in ensuring patients understand the information, when their native language is not used in the consent form. In certain circumstances, patients would prefer not to make decisions by themselves. They often wish to share decision-making with their family or physician and occasionally want others to make decisions on their behalf. Physicians should ask first who patients want to engage in the decision-making process and how they want to make decisions, rather than just what decision they want to make (Terry 2006).

In western culture, informed consent focuses on the principle of autonomy. As noted by Beauchamp and Childress: "A person's decision is autonomous if it comes from the person's values and beliefs, is based on adequate information and understanding, and is not determined by internal or external constraints that compel the decision" (Beauchamp and Childress 2013). The "four principles" of autonomy, beneficence, nonmaleficence, and justice, as proposed by Beauchamp and Childress (2013) are the foundation of a prevalent ethics framework used throughout of western cultures; however, the weight with which they are considered and their understanding differs in other cultures. Although the principle of autonomy is acknowledged in Islam, individual rights are restricted by Islamic law and there are certain differences in the understanding and applications of autonomy. Accordingly, the principle of autonomy does not bear the same weight as it does in many western cultures. Autonomy is only applicable for actions that are permissible; Islamic teachings assert that an individual should not inflict on himself, his own property, or honor any actions deemed forbidden, as the rights of God supersede individual rights (Chamsi-Pasha and Albar 2013a). Accordingly, physicians must give patients an opportunity of informed choice and the right of informed refusal. A patient must be aware of, understand, and accept the risks of refusing a proposed treatment and this should be documented.

Obtaining the patient's permission prior to delivering medical treatment is obligatory in Islam if the patient has full legal capacity or permission must be obtained from his legal guardian if the patient is a minor or incompetent. It should be noted that this is only if the treatment prescribed is permissible. According to the International Fiqh Academy (1992) however, consent is not required if the treatment and the medical procedures are needed in emergency situation to save a life or vital organs; when the patient is unconscious; or the patient is a minor, and no guardian is available; in cases of contagious diseases; and when preventive immunizations are ordered by the health authorities. Additionally, consent is not required if a minor's legal guardian refuses to give permission and it is clearly detrimental to the patient under his/her guardianship.

While this may be different to conventional law regarding medical practice, it is derived from the principles of *fiqh* (Islamic law), "harm should not be inflicted nor reciprocated" (*laa dharar'a wa laa dhiraar*), and "public interest should be prioritized over personal interest" (*al-maslahah al-aam tuqaddam 'alaa al-maslahah al-khassah*). If the treatment is obligated, refraining from treatment by a patient is an act of misconduct, and preventing misconduct is an obligation upon all Muslims (Sharifudin 2014). However, in terms of decision-making, it is important to mention that sometimes a patient may ask his doctor: "What is your advice in my condition? What would you do if your parent was in my situation?" The physician may feel embarrassed, but the physician should be honest and give sincere advice. The matter may be more complicated when the patient relegates the decision-making to his physician by saying: "I have trust in you, and whatever you decide I will accept." The physician should be tactful and explain that the decision should be in the hands of the patient and his family. He might help by reviewing all the necessary information, and perhaps give his personal advice. In cases where the patient does not want to know the diagnosis, the physician should make sure that the patient understands the information given to him, and may discuss the patient's condition with the family and let them try to persuade the patient to at least to take part in the decision-making. The question of confidentiality will crop up here if the family gets to know the details of the ailment and its management. In cases that the patient agrees to divulge the intricacies of his medical condition to the family or proxy, then there is no breaking of confidentiality, as it is done after getting the consent of the patient himself (Albar and Chamsi-Pasha 2015).

The process of informed consent is more complicated in clinical research, especially when the treating physician is conducting a clinical trial. Clinical investigators should be reminded that the informed consent document alone does not assure the subject's full understanding of their participation. It is important to make sure that the subjects understand and distinguish their treatment decisions from clinical research. Therefore, before the subject makes his decision, the research team should discuss the study purpose and procedures, risks and benefits, and the rights and obligations of the participant. If the subject decides then to participate, he will sign the consent form. Furthermore, once the subject decides to participate in the study, the research team should continue to draw the participant's attention to any new information that may affect his situation. Before, during, or after the study, subjects should also have the opportunity to ask questions and discuss any issues they may encounter. Thus, informed consent is a continuous process, rather than a single discussion point (Alahmad 2012; Chamsi-Pasha and Albar 2008).

However, when obtaining informed consent in situations that involve end-of-life decisions, the patient's values should be the focus, and the physician acts as an advisor, rather than an agent.

## Cross-Gender Considerations in the Physician–Patient Relationship

Gender roles, relationship dynamics, and boundaries are culture-specific, and are frequently shaped by religious teachings. Acknowledgement of the importance of cultural practices in patients' lives is required together with work to minimize the negative consequences of cultural differences in medical care (Padela and Rodriguez del Pozo 2011). For example, if you ask an American unmarried girl if she has a child, she would not be offended. However, if an unmarried Muslim girl is asked the same question she would be offended since an unmarried girl does not usually participate in relations outside of wedlock. The Qur'an recommends both men and women to "lower their gaze and guard their modesty" and further instructs women to "not display their beauty and ornaments except what (must ordinarily) appear thereof" (24: 30-31). A statement of the Prophet Muhammad goes further, "it does not suit (a woman past the age of menarche) that she displays her parts of body except this and this" pointing to the face and hands (Sunan Abu Dawud). These verses and multiple other Traditions from the Prophet (PBUH) form the basis of the Islamic dress code, specifically the regulations of the areas of the body that must be clothed (*awrah*). These regulations are intended to safeguard honor and dignity (Padela and Rodriguez del Pozo 2011). Muslim women often choose to cover their hair with a scarf called *hijab*, and it is essential that physicians respect it and allow them to do so whenever possible. For example, even when going to the operating room for surgery, it is preferable to allow a Muslim woman to wear her *hijab* in addition to the hospital gown. If this is not permitted, using a surgical head and neck covering can allow a woman to maintain her sense of comfort and dignity without compromising hospital and operating room policy (Hussain *et al.* 2010). When the patient gown is a necessity, hospital staff could offer to keep the curtains drawn, or the door closed, so that patients can be spared from onlookers. Another effective way is a "knock–wait–enter" policy by which staff knock, wait for permission and then enter patient rooms. It must be stressed that the clinician uncover only that part of the body that needs to be examined, and cover those parts that are not necessary to examine or have been examined already (Padela and Rodriguez del Pozo 2011).

Avoiding unnecessary exposure is an important priority. In the clinic, asking a Muslim woman to undress and put on examination shorts or a robe may be uncomfortable for her. Muslim women are encouraged to wear loose fitting clothing that can be stretched to allow adequate exposure for examination while maintaining as much coverage as possible. Although a patient may be unconscious, covering the genital area in the operating room with a surgical towel during skin preparation is also encouraged and conveys an additional element of respect and thus engenders trust between the patient and the surgeon (Hussain *et al.* 2010).

"*Khalwah*" is defined as the situation where a "man and a woman are both located in a closed place alone and where physical touch between them can occur." This situation is prohibited between adult members of opposite sexes (*non-mahram;* individuals who are not very close relatives or spouses), in order to prevent the accusation, or committal, of illicit relations. This prohibition stems from Prophetic traditions stating that "when a *non-mahram* male and a female are alone, Satan is the third among them" and also stating that "a man must not remain alone in the company of a woman" (Sahīh Al-Bukhārī 2012). Therefore, clinicians should also consider inviting a third person to attend during visits to avoid a situation where an unrelated man and a woman are alone.

A Muslim doctor examining a female patient must have a third party in the room (i.e. a nurse) in order to have a chaperone so that the issue of sexual harassment will not be a problem. Also, there is extreme sensitivity about maintaining the virginity of an unmarried Muslim girl, thus vaginal examination should only be the last resort for an unmarried girl (Hathout 2000). The Qur'an exhorts "Nor come nigh to adultery: for it is a shameful (deed) and an evil, opening the road (to other evils)" (17:32). Thus Islamic law not only prohibits adultery but also strictly regulates physical contact since the verse bars "proximity" to adultery.

In Islamic culture, both men and women are more sensitive about being naked. For instance, patients do not want to be examined while completely naked, so their interest, dignity and privacy should be considered. Most Islamic scholars believe that a patient seeking non-urgent treatment should choose a physician according to the following order of decreasing preference Muslim of the same gender, non-Muslim of the same gender, Muslim of the opposite gender, non-Muslim of the opposite gender (Padela 2011, Islamic Fiqh Academy 1993, Decree 81–12/8). If a male physician is professionally more experienced then he could take priority and the same would apply to a Muslim or non-Muslim physician.

A physician of the same faith is recommended based on the assumption that a Muslim physician would be able to advise the patient when medical treatment takes precedence over religious obligations. However, it is important to note that Islamic law does allow for deviation from normal regulations in cases of necessity and emergency.

For instance, Ibn Muflih, of the Hanbali school states: "If a woman is sick and no female doctor is available, a male doctor may treat her. In such a case, the doctor is permitted to examine her, including her genitalia." Scholars are also clear that female doctors may fully examine male patients in cases of necessity. In all cases, a third party of the same gender as the patient is required to be present for the examination (Aldeen 2007). A provider holding the hand of a patient who just lost a family member may be viewed as a boundary crossing by some and compassionate by others. Some Muslim women choose not to shake hands with unrelated males, even in the context of business and healthcare. This abstinence is not a sign of disrespect but is simply an expression of a Muslim woman's display of her belief. The doctor may ask a Muslim woman how she would like to be greeted and this can avoid potential embarrassment for the patient and misunderstanding by the doctor (Hussain 2010). Physical contact outside of the examination should always be approached with caution. Understanding a Muslim woman's concerns about modesty is invaluable in developing an appropriate physician–patient relationship.

## Confidentiality in Physician–Patient Relationships

Confidentiality is an important concept in Islam based on three Islamic principles: first, the prohibition of backbiting (*fitnah*), as mentioned in Qur'an: "neither backbite one another" (49:12); second, the duty to protect secrets; and third, the consideration of the protection of confidentiality as a kind of loyalty, which has to be saved from harm (Alahmad 2012). A number of revelation texts in the Qur'an and *hadith* emphasize the importance of avoiding negative conversations about other people in their absence (backbiting) even if the facts discussed are true and even after they have died. This is based on several Qur'anic verses; "Those who are faithfully true to their *amanât* (all the duties which Allâh has ordained, honesty, moral responsibility and trust) and to their covenants" (23:8). In a *fatwa* issued in 1993 by the International Islamic Fiqh Academy, jurists affirmed that a breach of confidentiality can be acceptable only if the harm of maintaining confidentiality overrides its benefits. This *fatwa* is the most important *fatwa* to deal with confidentiality and clearly states the obligation of maintaining medical confidentiality in the medical profession. Moreover, it elucidates some situations in which breaching confidentiality is allowed or mandatory (Alahmad 2012).

Medical confidentiality is one of the basic components in building a trusting PPR. Keeping a patient's secrets and maintaining confidentiality is both a legal and ethical duty. However, disclosure of such secrets is permitted in different legal systems such as notification of births and deaths, infectious diseases, child abuse, medical errors, drug side effects and dangerous pregnancies (Milanifar *et al.* 2014). Muslim physicians keep the secrets of the patient, his family and even his servants, whom the physician encounters while visiting the patient at his home. This attitude is also part of benefiting the patient (beneficence) and not doing any harm to him (non-maleficence). However, if divulging the secret may be of benefit to the patient, as considered by his physician, then it should be exposed, as far as it benefits him or wards off potential harm.

Therefore, if breaking confidentiality can prevent harm, e.g. if a psychiatric patient tells his doctor that he is going to kill a person (due to delusions and hallucinations), then the psychiatrist has a duty to inform the police and also to inform the person to be attacked, so that he may take steps to avoid being attacked. However, the physicians should be aware of reciprocal reaction in tribal areas. In case of a HIV-positive patient, a physician has a duty to inform his spouse of the true diagnosis (i.e. HIV). In practice, he should obtain permission to disclose from the infected person, or require the patient to tell his spouse in the physician's presence of the true diagnosis; otherwise he would be allowing harm to occur to the spouse. The Islamic Fiqh Academy issued a decree in 1995 stating that: "Deliberately infecting a healthy individual with HIV (AIDS) in any form of deliberate work is forbidden (*haram*)." If the health authorities require reporting infectious diseases then it should be reported so that measures may be taken to protect the whole community; and breaking confidentiality in such cases is allowed. If the magistrate orders the physician to divulge the true diagnosis, in most cases he must obey, lest he would be accused of obstructing justice (Albar and Chamsi-Pasha 2015).

Visual recording of patients and human subjects is commonly used for clinical and research purposes. It is most prevalent in the specialties of plastic surgery, wound care, otolaryngology, dermatology, and maxillofacial surgery. Images are also commonly used for academic purposes, including publication, training healthcare professionals, and educating the public. The judicial system can require recordings as evidence of an alleged assault as well. The literature suggests that there are both detrimental and favorable effects of recording human subjects. In order to regulate these activities, several practice standards regarding biomedical recording have been issued by certain health authorities, professional associations and journals (Saidun 2013).

Muslim jurists' rulings on medical recording vary from permission to discouragement to prohibition. However, the ruling is ultimately dependent on the purpose of the recording, the intended use of the images, the way in which the recording session is conducted, the type of images captured, and the potential consequences of the whole experience. For images to be deemed permissible, all of the aforementioned circumstances must not contradict *Shari'a* law.

In order to maintain a healthy relationship with subjects, researchers must provide to subjects an explanation about the recording, including the purpose, process, withdrawal of consent, confidentiality and use of the images. Written consent should be obtained from the patient or his/her legal representatives before the procedure. The patient's rights and dignity must be respected, taking into consideration their cultural and religious background. Only the minimum necessary area should be photographed. Images should be securely stored, with access restricted to authorized personnel with justified reasons for viewing the images. The Islamic code of conduct must be observed during the recording sessions, where the rules of modesty and cross-gender interaction apply. Conventional standards strongly recommend the use of a chaperone in the presence of semi- or fully-naked subjects of the opposite sex, while the Islamic standard obligates the use of chaperones whenever a photographer is dealing with a subject of the opposite sex in an enclosed space, regardless of the extent and area of exposure (Saidun 2013).

## Disclosure and Breaking Bad News in Physician–Patient Relationships

In Islamic societies, one of the challenging decisions for clinicians is whether to disclose information to the patient, or to conceal it from the patient and disclose it to the family instead. The impact of true diagnosis on the patient depends largely on how it is told. The patient can be prepared by choosing the right time, revealing the news gradually, showing empathy and concern, concentrating on what is more distressing to the patient, i.e. pain, death, and so on, and softening the news. For instance, a physician might say: nobody knows exactly; healthy people die for non-medical reasons; life doesn't end here; you have a chance to put your affairs in order, which is an opportunity that a lot of people don't have. It may be impossible to conceal the information from the patient for an extended period of time. As mentioned earlier, the relationship should be based on honesty, trust and respect for the patient's autonomy as well as beneficence to the patient. Disclosure to the patient would improve trust in physicians in general and relieve the family from the burden of breaking the bad news to the patient. However, patients react differently when being told that they have a terminal illness and in some cases disclosure to the patient may cause undue distress to the patient and may even lead to suicide. It is important that a physician balance the harm versus the benefit and be prepared for such reactions from their patients. An ethical dilemma physicians frequently face, is informing patients about their terminal illness, or an incurable disease that is expected to result in death within a short period of time. Disclosure of such crucial information to the patient can be considered harmful by the physician and/or patient's family. On the other hand, not telling the patient the truth or revealing it to the family without his/her permission violates the patient's rights of autonomy and confidentiality. The decision to disclose terminal illness information is complex but usually centers on disagreements about the limits of paternalism (on part of the physician and/or the family), and the proper balance between the physician's duty of beneficence to the patient and the patient's right to autonomy and confidentiality. In Islamic societies it has been accepted that a physician can withhold information from the patient if he has good reason to believe that divulging the information to that patient is going to cause harm, impair management, or cause distress.

However, this should be documented in the patient's file and the consent of the substitute decision-maker or legal representative should be obtained.

Breaking bad news is one of the most distressing tasks faced by physicians on daily basis; however, not all physicians receive formal training on breaking bad news. Bad news is "any information likely to alter drastically a patient's view of his or her future." It can range from the need to undergo further laboratory or radiological investigations to confirm the diagnosis, to informing the patient of a life-threatening disease such as cancer, or informing the family or friends of a major morbidity or death of their loved ones (Salem and Salem 2013).

The concern about breaking bad news is due to the strong impact on both patients and physicians. Furthermore, clinicians who feel inadequately trained in communication skills have significantly higher distress levels when faced with patients' suffering. An appropriate delivery of bad news is, in turn, associated with increased patient satisfaction (Martins and Carvalho 2013). Han and Kagan pointed out that "we do not adequately teach patient communication in medical training. This real-world skill is probably more important to a physician's performance than technical proficiencies. Talking to patients about death is quite hard and, unlike learning other medical skills, it does not become easier with repetition. Every encounter with a dying patient is unique and once the physician believes he has found the 'formula' to appropriately delivering bad news, he quickly discovers that one size does not fit all" (Han and Kagan 2013). However, several problems arise when physicians break bad news; some of which are specific to Muslim countries. Breaking bad news would ideally require lengthy preparation and adequate time. In practice, due to patient overload, time is a luxury which many physicians in Muslim countries do not possess. Besides, physicians practicing in Muslim countries require culture-specific training to break bad news and this is not currently incorporated into the medical curriculum in the majority of developing countries (Tavakol 2008).

The majority of patients in developed countries prefer to know their diagnosis, options of treatment, adverse effects, and prognosis of their malignant disease. The codes of ethics of a number of Asian and Eastern countries require that any fatal diagnosis or prognosis first be disclosed to a family member. Following discussion with the treating physician, the family judges whether communicating the truth is in the best interests of the patient. The truth is often concealed for fear that it will extinguish the patient's hopes, leading to desperation, physical suffering, anxiety, and a hastened death (de Pentheny O'Kelly *et al.* 2011). Most families then tend to withhold crucial information that — based on their best knowledge — might lead to psychological suffering of their loved ones. Physicians working in Muslim communities are required to balance between the patient's rights to be informed with the relative's request to avoid emotionally upsetting the patient. Thus, physicians must tailor the amount and detail of the information about bad news based on the patient's desire (Tavakol 2008). The physician may withhold the information from the patient if he feels that disclosing the information to the patient is going to cause him harm or unbearable distress.

The physician should ask the patient for approval of the attendance of family and friends during the encounter for breaking the bad news. He should conduct the interview in a sizable, private room to allow enough space for desired attendees. Bad news should be disclosed in simple and clear terms that match the educational level of the patient without going into many details. During the meeting the physician should pay special attention to the body language of the patient and his/her family. Is the patient afraid, stressed, or at ease? Does the patient have a religious background? In patients who have strong religious views, physicians should stress the positive and optimistic religious statements such as, "everything is in the hands of God." In patients who prefer a non-disclosure approach, physicians are encouraged to stress a paternalistic approach such as "don't worry, we will do everything possible to improve your health" or "you're in good hands" (Salem and Salem 2013). If the patient opts for a substitute decision-maker role for a partner or a family member, then breaking bad news would be directed to the substitute decision-maker. Patients or family members should be encouraged to ask questions and the interview should be ended with supportive and empathic statements.

## Conclusion

The concept of an effective, trusting PPR is one of the major issues in providing healthcare throughout the world. Unfortunately PPRs have slipped nowadays, in many circumstances, into more consumer-like relationships. Consequently, the level of trust between physicians and their patients has been somehow tarnished. Islamic teachings encourage Muslims to seek treatment; and medical practice is considered a sacred duty in Islam, with physicians being rewarded by God for their proper work. Physicians should be aware that Muslims' faith in God helps them cope with their disease. The character traits required of the virtuous physician are already embedded in the Qur'an and the *Sunna*. The Muslim physician, guided by these two major sources of Islamic law, will cultivate the necessary character of a good physician. The physician must be pure in character, diligent, and conscientious in caring for his patients. Good practices include: respecting the modesty of patients and not requiring them to be completely naked when being examined; and taking the patient's medical history in private. The physician should ensure that a chaperone is present when a Muslim male doctor examines a female patient. A physician may withhold information from the patient if he has good reason to believe that divulging the information to that patient will cause harm, impair management of the disease, or cause distress. Healthcare providers need to be knowledgeable about these religious and cultural factors to be able to provide culturally-competent healthcare. Continuing professional development and education is required to ensure that physicians see their patients as persons, and not as a diseased organ.

## References

Alahmad, G. and Dierickx, K. 2012. What Do Islamic Institutional *Fatwas* Say About Medical and Research Confidentiality and Breach of Confidentiality? *Developing World Bioethics* 12(2), 104–12.

Albar, M. A. and Chamsi-Pasha, H. 2015. *Contemporary Bioethics: Islamic Perspective.* New York: Springer.

Aldeen, A. Z. 2007. The Muslim Ethical Tradition and Emergent Medical Care: An Uneasy Fit. *Academic Emergency Medicine* 14(3), 277–8.

Arawi, T. A. 2011. The Ethics of the Muslim Physician and the Legacy of Muhammad (PBUH). *Journal of the Islamic Medical Association of North America* 43, 35–8.

Balint, M. 1957. *The Doctor, His Patient and the Illness*. Edinburgh: Churchill Livingstone. In: Meza, J. P. and Fahoome, G. F. 2008. The Development of an Instrument for Measuring Healing. *Annals of Family Medicine* 6, 355–60.

Banerjee, A. and Sanyal, D. 2012. Dynamics of Doctor–Patient Relationship: A Cross-Sectional Study on Concordance, Trust, and Patient Enablement. *Journal Family Community Medicine* 19, 12–9.

Beauchamp, T. L. and Childress, J. F. 2013. *Principles of Biomedical Ethics*. 7th ed. New York: Oxford University Press.

Chamsi-Pasha, H. and Albar, M. A. 2008. *Akhlakiyat al-Bohouth al-Tebia'a* [Medical Research Ethics]. Damascus: Dar al-Kalam.

Chamsi-Pasha, H. and Albar, M. A. 2013a. Western and Islamic Bioethics: How Close is the Gap? *Avicenna Journal of Medicine* 3(1), 8–14.

Chamsi-Pasha, H. and Albar, M. A. 2013b. Islamic Medical Ethics a Thousand Years Ago. *Saudi Medical Journal* 34(7), 673–5.

de Pentheny O'Kelly, C., Urch, C.; Brown, E. A. 2011. The Impact of Culture and Religion on Truth Telling at the End of Life. *Nephrology Dialysis and Transplantation* 26(12), 3838–42.

Frey, J. J. 3rd. 2013. Communication as Prevention: The Value of Talking with Each Other. *World Medical Journal* 112(4), 156–7.

Halligan, P. 2006. Caring for Patients of Islamic Denomination: Critical Care Nurses' Experiences in Saudi Arabia. *Journal of Clinical Nursing* 15, 1565–73.

Han, J. and Kagan, A. R. 2012. Breaking Bad News. *American Journal of Clinical Oncology* 35(4), 309–10.

Hathout, H. 2000. Medical Ethics: An Islamic Point of View. Available at: http://www.drhassanhathout.org/medicalethics/medical_ethics_an_islamic_point_of_view.html. [Last visited January 4, 2016].

Hussain, W., Hussain, H., Hussain, M., Hussain, S. and Attar, S. 2010. Approaching the Muslim Orthopedic Patient. *Journal of Bone and Joint Surgery, American Volume* 92(7), e2.

Islam, M. S. and Jhora, S. T. 2012. Physician–Patient Relationship: The Present Situation and Our Responsibilities. *Bangladesh Medical Journal* 41(1), 55–58.

Islamic Code of Medical Ethics. 1981. First International Conference on Islamic Medicine held in Kuwait at the onset of the 15th Hijri Century (6–10 Rabie A wal 1401: 12–16 January, 1981).

Martins, R. G. and Carvalho, I. P. 2013. Breaking Bad News: Patients' Preferences And Health Locus of Control. *Patient Education and Counseling* 92(1), 67–73.

Milanifar, A., Larijani, B., Paykarzadeh, P., Ashtari, G. and Akhondi M. M. 2014. Breaching Confidentiality: Medical Mandatory Reporting Laws in Iran. *Journal of Medical Ethics and History of Medicine* 7, 13.

Ott B. B., Al-Khadhuri, J. and Al-Junaibi, S. 2003. Preventing Ethical Dilemmas: Understanding Islamic Healthcare Practices. *Pediatrc Nursing* 29, 227–30.

Packer, S. 2011. Informed Consent with a Focus on Islamic Views. *Journal of the Islamic Medical Association of North America* 43, 215–8.

Padela, A. I. and Rodriguez del Pozo, P. 2011. Muslim Patients and Cross-Gender Interactions in Medicine: An Islamic Bioethical Perspective. *Journal of Medical Ethics* 37(1), 40–4.

Rhazes, A. B. 2001. *Akhlaq al-Tabib* [Medical Ethics]. Ed. Al-Abd AL. Cairo: Dar Al-Turath, 130–3.

Sahih Al Bukhari. 2002. *Dar Al-Risalah*. Beirut, Lebanon.

Saidun, S. 2013. Photographing Human Subjects in Biomedical Disciplines: An Islamic Perspective. *Journal of Medical Ethics* 39(2), 84–8.

Salem, A., Salem, A. F. 2013. Breaking Bad News: Current Prospective and Practical Guideline For Muslim Countries. *Journal of Cancer Education* 28(4), 790–4.

Sharifudin, M. A., Wan Husin, W. R. and Taib, M. N. 2014. Religious Perspective of Doctor–Patient Relationship Models in Complementing Uprising Social Phenomenal Demands. *Abstract of Emerging Trends in Scientific Research* 1, 1–10.

Tavakol, M., Murphy, R. and Torabi, S. 2008. Educating Doctors About Breaking Bad News: An Iranian Perspective. *Journal of Cancer Education* 23(4), 260–3.

Terpstra, O. T. 2012. On Doctor–Patient Relationship and Feedback Interventions. *Perspectives on Medical Education* 1, 159–61.

Terry, P. B. 2006. Informed Consent in Clinical Medicine. *Chest* 26, 575–82.

# CHAPTER SIX

## Islamic Perspective on Brain Death
## and Organ Transplantation

### *Abul Fadl Mohsin Ebrahim*

### Summary

Death of the vast majority of human beings is still being determined upon the cessation of heartbeat and respiration. A body that becomes lifeless is in no position to breathe nor can it move. In other words it does not manifest any of the signs of life. However, modern biotechnological innovation has made it possible for patients with head injuries, for example, who are unable to breathe on their own, to do so by means of a ventilator. It is in such cases that the problem of determining the moment of death arises. Muslim scholars have always been concerned about ascertaining the end of human life because of the worldly and religious consequences that follow the pronouncement of death.

This chapter includes the insights of Muslim scholars on the moment of death and the retrieval of organs from brainstem-dead patients. Additionally, the opinions of some prominent Muslim jurists, both for and against the issue of utilizing human organs, are explored together with guidelines proposed by Muslim jurists based on the original sources of Islam, namely, the Qur'an and *Sunna* (Prophetic tradition) as well Islamic juridical principles. Furthermore, this chapter also makes reference to resolutions taken by the various Islamic Juridical Academies on this issue and the validity of including organ donation in one's will.

## Introduction

Organs that can be donated are the heart, intestines, kidneys, liver, lungs, and pancreas. Tissues that can be donated include corneas, heart valves, and skin. Such donations may benefit people who have organ failure; who are blind; who have severe burns; or are suffering from serious diseases. As human beings, we are all aware of the fact that before the inevitable strikes, some of us could be afflicted with diseases which may necessitate medical care and attention. Most times we are able to overcome our ailments by resting, taking relevant medications, observing an appropriate diet, etc. However, we cannot rule out the possibility that at some point in life one of our organs could cease to function. If this were to happen, depending on the nature of the damage, we would have to undergo corrective surgery or have the defective organ replaced altogether.

Replacing diseased or damaged organs is not a modern innovation. Jeff Zhorne (1985, 10) points out that, as early as the 8th century BC, Hindu surgeons performed skin transplants to replace noses lost due to syphilis, physical combat, or punishment for crimes. Likewise, in the *hadith* literature, we come across the incident of Ufrajah, a Companion (*sahabi*) of the Prophet, who lost his nose during a battle and had it replaced with an artificial one made out of silver. His silver nose soon gave rise to poor smell and he sought the advice of the Prophet who counseled him to have another made out of gold (*Sunan Abi Dawud* 2:92). However, transplantation of an organ from the same species was not achieved until 1913 when Alexis Carrel, a French surgeon, succeeded in transplanting a kidney from one cat to another. This became possible only after he had mastered the sewing of severed blood vessels end to end, enabling them to carry blood as efficiently as they had before the operation (Zhorne 1985, 11). Thereafter, in the early 1950s, an orthotopic heart transplant in a dog was carried out.

In preparation for the first ever human heart transplant, Christiaan Barnard and his team of surgeons performed heart transplants in dogs and a kidney transplant on a Mrs. Black. Subsequently, on 3 December 1967, Barnard and his South African surgical team made history by transplanting the heart of Denise Darvall, a 24-year-old woman, certified brain dead after involvement in a motor vehicle accident, into 54-year-old Louis Washkansky. Washkansky lived for 18 days and died as a result of a lung infection which led to the weakening of the heart from lack of oxygen. About a year later, on the 2 January 1968, Barnard performed yet another heart transplant. The recipient of the donor heart was Dr Philip Blaiberg, a Cape Town dental surgeon, who eventually left the hospital to return to full active life. Commenting on his patient's amazing recovery, Barnard (1987, xx) wrote: "His courage and fortitude did much to establish heart transplantation as a realistic option for future patients with terminal heart disease."

Insofar as tissue and organ transplantation itself is concerned one must bear in mind that the Qur'an and *Sunna* neither sanction it nor condemn it. Contemporary Muslim jurists have deliberated on the issue and proposed certain juristic guidelines based on their deductions from the broad teachings of the two original sources of *Shari'a*, namely, the Qur'an and *Sunna*. Thus, as in all matters which are not categorically addressed in these two original sources, differences of opinion among Muslim jurists surface on the issue of organ transplantation. The problems that organ transplantation poses to the Muslim mind may be summarized as follows: firstly, a Muslim believes that whatever he owns or possesses has been given to him in trust (*amanah*) from Allah. Some consider it a breach of trust to give consent for the removal of parts from one's body, while still alive, for transplantation to benefit another person. Secondly, the Islamic law (*Shari'a*) emphasizes the sacredness of the human body. Some consider it an act of aggression against the human body tantamount to mutilation if organs are removed after death for the purpose of transplantation. Thirdly, since the most viable organs for transplantation are from patients who have been diagnosed as brain dead, some would consider it an act of murder to remove their organs for transplantation purposes.

Throughout the world, the number of people needing organ transplants far exceeds the available supply and thousands die while they wait helplessly for an organ. This has prompted some countries to adopt certain policies to assure the availability of organs for transplantation. Crowe and Cohen (2006) point out that most of the American states have "first person consent" laws in respect of organ donation. This therefore gives paramountcy to the individual person's decision whether or not to donate his/her organs. Thus a living individual, who wishes to donate a "non-essential" organ, is entitled to do so as long as he understands the risks and benefits of donation and is medically eligible to donate. This is in line with the views of Muslims scholars who justify organ donation. Zahir (undated, 85). Mason (1999, 343) mentions that in the United Kingdom, according to common law, living donations prohibit a person consenting to being killed or seriously injured. The late Sheikh Jad al-Haqq (1994, 428) concurs that a Muslim too cannot donate any of his vital organs while still being alive. As for cadaveric donation, in the absence of that person's formal consent prior to his/her demise, then someone close to that person could give consent for the removal of tissue for organ for transplantation purposes (Mason 1999, 342). However, Tanzil-ur-Rahman (1980), contends that for a Muslim who stipulates in his will that his organ may be used for transplantation into someone else's body, the transplantation would only be effected if none of his heirs raise any objection to that directive. According to Montgomery (2003), retrieving tissues and organs from brainstem-dead patients is contingent upon their having given their consent and that the diagnosis for brainstem death ought to have been done by two doctors who are independent of the transplant team, and that at least one of them should be a consultant. In the absence of the patient's consent, then consent from a close relative should be sought. In the Muslim world, Mahmoud Tabatabaei (2014, 65) rightly points out that to date there is no consensus on brain death as the determinant factor for the moment of death since, according to the Qur'an, human death occurs when the soul departs the body which is in effect consistent with irreversible cessation of all signs of human life and not just the brain's functions.

## Brain Death

In the past, death was considered to be a simple and straightforward phenomenon. The general practitioner would issue the death certificate once he was convinced that there was cessation or absence of spontaneous life in the patient. This meant that the patient had stopped breathing, his heart had stopped beating, there was unresponsiveness, his body had turned cold and, finally, rigor mortis had set in (Ebrahim and Haffejee 1989).

With the successful accomplishment of heart transplantation, it became obvious that determining the moment of death required further thought.

Cessation of heartbeat is no longer considered evidence of death since the heart can now be substituted with that of a just-deceased donor or with that of a baboon or even with a mechanical one. Moreover, modern biomedical innovations like the resuscitator and cardiac pacemaker have made it imperative to establish a set of criteria by which the moment of death can be identified (Häring 1972).

Frank Ayd describes death as "an orderly progression from clinical death to brain death, to biological death, to cellular death" and elucidates the progression as follows: clinical death occurs "when the body's vital functions — respiration and heartbeat — wane and finally cease." Clinical death may in some cases be reversed. For example, a child who has drowned and is pulled out of water without heartbeat and respiration can be saved through the initiation of mouth-to-mouth resuscitation and cardiac massage. Brain death occurs after cardiac and respiratory arrest because "under normal temperature conditions, the human brain cannot survive loss of oxygen for more than 10 minutes." As a result of anoxia, the component parts of the brain die in progressive steps. Death of the cortex is followed by that of the midbrain and finally ending with the brainstem. When the whole brain has died, biological death takes place. Biological death is denoted by the absence of bodily movements. A dead brain cannot sustain bodily life. Once bodily life ceases, cellular death follows (Lyons 1970).

From the above, it is clear that death occurs progressively and that death of the brain is the determining factor in the process of dying. Ahmad Elkadi (1989, 361), aptly explains that:

> Any other organ may die or be surgically removed and yet the owner continues to live, retaining his reason, power of thinking, awareness, personality, and everything else, either because the organ concerned is one that a person can live without such as the limbs, parts of the stomach, or the intestines and so on, or because of the availability of a replacement which can carry on the functions of that organ for a long or short period of time.

However, the brain is a different kind of organ altogether. The brain cells, as Harmon L. Smith (1970) points out, are extremely sensitive to anoxia. Thus cerebral cortical cells begin to die within five minutes if deprived of oxygenated blood, and death of the whole brain results thereafter within approximately the next 10 minutes. The other vital organs like the heart, for example, can be reactivated after several minutes of cessation; the kidneys can still be viable after the lapse of one hour following nephrectomy; and corneal transplants can still be carried out although several days may have elapsed since they were surgically removed. Moreover, unlike other vital organs, the brain cannot be replaced in view of the fact that a sound living brain can only be found in a living person and there is no substitute for the human brain in the foreseeable future. For this reason modern medical science holds that brain death determines the end of human life. This is confirmed in a statement made by Goulon and Babinet: "The brain only gives man his reality; where it has disappeared, man no longer is. Such is also the opinion expressed by the leading national and international medical authorities" (Häring 1972).

Furthermore, the observation made by Mukhtar al-Mahdi (1989), a neurosurgeon, may be relevant to the understanding of brain death:

> Damaged brain cells are irreplaceable. But by resorting to the ventilator, the organs of the body other than the brain may be kept alive for a period of time ranging from a few hours to two weeks, more or less. But that period cannot go on much longer even if we continue to give the patient all the stimulating aids possible. Blood pressure would begin to drop, food assimilation processes would slow down, body temperature would drop, and finally the heart would stop.

It is important to point out here that a vegetative state should not be confused with the diagnosis of brain death. Vegetative patients are able to breathe spontaneously; at times they can follow objects with their eyes; they do respond to painful stimuli; and in due course may even recover from their neurological disability. Thus patients suffering from irreversible coma are certified brain dead only after stringent tests have been carried out on them. These tests will confirm the patients' unresponsiveness to painful stimuli; their pupils' non-reaction to light and remaining fixed and dilated; their inability to swallow, yawn or vocalize; and their inability to breathe spontaneously within a three-minute period after the ventilator is switched off. A flat electroencephalogram (EEG) will further verify the absence of electric waves being transmitted by the brain. Extreme caution is taken before finally pronouncing such patients brain dead. These clinical examinations are repeated at regular intervals to ensure that there is no improvement in the patients' condition (Ebrahim and Haffejee 1989, 9). In the event that organ donation is envisaged, upon confirmation of brain death diagnosis, the patients are reconnected to the ventilator, and kept in the intensive therapy unit (ITU) until the transplant surgery can be carried out (Evans 1993, 136). Vital organs, for example, heart, lungs, kidneys, and liver of brain dead patients have a better chance of functioning in the post-operative period. This, however, should not lead us to believe that the motivation behind declaring patients to be brain dead is conditioned by the interest of transplant surgeons to harvest the organs for transplantation purposes. As a matter of fact, physicians who are to be associated with the subsequent organ transplantation are precluded from making the diagnosis of brain death (Ebrahim and Haffejee 1989, 9).

### Insights on the Moment of Death

Al-Ghazali (undated, Vol. 4), explains that death occurs at the moment when the soul is separated from the body and that at this juncture the body ceases to be an instrument of the soul. Muslim jurists in general uphold the traditional definition of clinical death which is permanent cessation of heart beat and respiration. However, as pointed out earlier, advances made in the field of biomedical technology have complicated the issue of determining the moment of death. The mechanical ventilator, for example, can help to keep the organs of the person diagnosed brain dead perfused with blood in order that these organs remain viable for transplantation. The issue of the moment of death is not regarded by Muslims as an amoral one; rather, it poses a real moral dilemma. In view of the fact that the Qur'an and the *Sunna* are silent on the issue of the brain death, there are differences of opinion among contemporary Muslim scholars.

Muslim physicians like Ahmad Shawqi Ibrahim and Ahmad Elkadi hold the view that the person whose brainstem has died may be pronounced dead (1989, 348 and 363). On the other hand, we find that there are Muslim physicians, like Hassan Hathout, who are cautious on pronouncing death upon a person whose brainstem has died. Hathout was of the view that, with the progress being made in the field of medical science, it may well be possible in the near or distant future to save the life of such a person (Mazkur 1989, 516).

Muslim jurists like Qadi Mujahid al-Islam Qasmi (1988, 5:14) state that "once the brainstem dies, the soul leaves the body." Likewise, Yasin (1989, 389–90) is of the opinion that "if damage to the brain is full and it [the brain] fails to respond to the soul's will and all other organs irrevocably fail, then the soul departs from the body by the will of Allah". There are other Muslim religious scholars holding the view that it would not be quite right to deem a person dead who has been diagnosed brain dead based on the following Islamic juridical principles:

(i) "what is known to be certain cannot be cancelled on the basis of what is suspected"; and
(ii) "the natural thing is for what has been to go on until a change is proved to have taken place" (Ardughdu 1989, 468).

Principle (ii) can be substantiated in the following statement of Al-Nawawi who suggests that death must be ascertained beyond any doubt:

> If there is suspicion of something unnatural about the death of a person, or if there is the possibility that it is a temporary failure, or if his face reveals signs of terror or something similar suggesting the possibility that he has fainted or that he is in a coma, or the like, (his burial) must be postponed until death is ascertained through the change of odour or something of that sort (Al-Wa'il 1989, 445).

In Kuwait, the Religious Rulings Committee of the Ministry of Endowment resolved on December 14, 1981 that a person cannot be considered dead when his brain has died as long as his respiration and circulation systems are alive, even if that life continues through mechanical aid (Al-Ashqar 1989, 402–403). However, Shaykh Badr al-Mutawalli Abd al-Basit and `Abd al-Qadir ibn Muhammad al-Amari (1989, 417 and 458) do not dismiss the probability that in the future Allah may inspire some researchers to discover a means to restore life to the brain after it has stopped functioning. Shaykh Muhammad al-Mukhtar al-Salami (1989, 422–423) is of the view that it would not be right to consider a brain dead person to be dead, as long as the essential systems of such a person are alive. It is however, important to note that the stance of contemporary Muslim scholars who are against endorsing brain death as the end of human life is based upon the view of the classical Muslim jurists who, as Tawfiq al-Wa'il (1989, 445) points out, never recognized the mind or awareness as the source of life but maintained that it is the body which is involved in determining life and death, because it is the body that actually moves.

## Retrieving Organs from Brain Dead Patients

Diagnosis of brainstem death is relevant to the issue of retrieving vital organs for transplantation purposes. In this regard, David Lamb (1993, 131) points out that "the most suitable cadaveric donors are brainstem dead individuals who have died in intensive care units."

Muslim scholars are divided on the issue of retrieving organs from brain dead patients for transplantation purposes. As for retrieving organs from brain death patients, there is no unanimity on the issue. Qadi Mujahid al-Islam (1988, 5:15) and the Muslim Judicial Council (undated), in Cape Town, South Africa, concur that further research needs to be undertaken on the issue of removing organs from brainstem-dead patients for transplantation purposes. The Council of Islamic Fiqh Academy of Organization of the Islamic Conference, during its fourth session held in Jeddah (1988), resolved that it is permissible to transplant the organ from a dead person to a living recipient on the condition that it has been authorized by the deceased or by his heirs after his death. The Council during the same session also noted that death may take two forms:

(i) when all functions of the brain come to a complete stop, and no medical cure can reverse the situation; or
(ii) when the heart and respiration come to a stop, and no medical cure can reverse the situation.

From the above, it may be implied, although not categorically stated, that it is permissible to retrieve organs from brain dead patients for transplantation purposes.

Mustafa Sabri Ardughdu (1989, 468) is of the view that if a just and trustworthy Muslim doctor is certain that the person whose heart or eye is to be removed is going to die soon it would then be lawful to transplant his organ to another person who is in need of it. Ardughdu bases his stance on the juridical principle which maintains that the right of the living supersedes consideration over that of the dead. Sheikh Muhammad al-Mukhtar al Salami (1989, 428), the former Mufti of Tunisia, states that "if a person is living only with the aid of resuscitation equipment, it is lawful to use his organ to save the life of another." He even stipulates that family members of such a person from whose body the organ is removed may waive their right to blood money. This implies that engaging in such a procedure is not to be regarded as a crime.

In the recommendations adopted at the conclusion of the Seminar on Human Life: Its Inception and End as Viewed by Islam, Kuwait, 1985, no mention was made of the permissibility of retrieving organs from brain-stem-dead patients, hence it remains an unresolved issue. Likewise, since the Council of Islamic Fiqh Academy of *Rabitat al-`Alam al Islami*, during its 10th session (1987), resolved that a person who is diagnosed brain dead can only be pronounced dead when respiration and heartbeat cease after switching off the life-support equipment, it *ipso facto* implies that retrieving organs from brainstem-dead patients is not permissible within the dictates of the *Shari'a*. In Cape Town, South Africa, the Muslim Judicial Council subscribes to the view that a person placed on a ventilator, whose heartbeat, circulation, and breathing are being kept going artificially, is to be considered alive. From this, it can be deduced that the Muslim Judicial Council is inclined towards the view that it would not be permissible to retrieve organs from brainstem-dead patients. In a document issued by the Majlis al-Ulama of Port Elizabeth, South Africa (1994), it is stated that removing any organs from a person pronounced brain dead entails two major crimes, namely, the perpetration of murder and perpetrating the unlawful act of misappropriating his organs.

## Deliberations of Muslim Scholars Against Organ Transplantation

Two prominent Muslim scholars who articulated their views against organ transplantation are Mufti Muhammad Shafi of Pakistan and Abd al-Salam al-Sukri of Egypt. Mufti Shafi holds organ transplantation not to be permissible on the basis of the following norms: sacredness of human life/body; the human body being an *amanah* (trust); and finally that such a procedure would be tantamount to subjecting the human body to material ends (Shafi 1967, 29–38).

These norms may be thus elucidated:

*Sacredness of human life and body*: From the teachings of the Qur'an it can be deduced that human beings are enjoined to protect and preserve their own lives as well as that of others. For example, they are forbidden from ending their own lives: "Do not kill or (destroy) yourselves: For verily Allah has been to you Most Merciful" (4:29), and also, "Make not your hands contribute to your own destruction" (2:195).

Likewise, the Qur'an imbues in every human being the gravity of a sin for taking someone else's life, as it states: "If anyone slays a human being, unless it be in legal punishment for murder or for spreading corruption on earth, it shall be as if he had slain the whole of mankind; whereas if anyone saves a life, it shall be as if he had saved the life of all mankind" (5:32).

In the *hadith* literature it is recorded that Prophet Muhammad made the following declaration in his farewell sermon (*Khutbat al Wada`ah*): "Your life and your property and your honour are sacred until you meet your Lord" (Da`wah-o-Irshad 1979).

The abovementioned citations have led Muslim jurists to include any form of aggression that is directed, not only against the life of a human being, but also against parts of his/her body as a crime (Awdah, 2:5). This view also gains support from the following *hadith*, "Breaking the bone of a dead person is equal in sinfulness and aggression to breaking it while a person is alive (*Sunan Abi Dawud. Hadith* no. 3207, 2:212–3).

In light of the above *hadith* the following questions may rightly be asked: How can one, therefore, be permitted to cut up a person's body and remove an organ from it? Would that not constitute an act of aggression against the human body and be tantamount to mutilation?

*The human body as an amanah (trust)*: The Qur'an (17:70; 21:20), tells us that Allah honoured humans, made serviceable to them whatever is on earth and in the heavens as a blessing and mercy. Likewise, it also mentions that Allah endowed humans with all that they need in respect of bodily organs (90:8). This understanding leads one to infer that humans have no right to donate any of their organs since these organs are not in reality their own, but have rather been given to them as an *amanah* (trust).

*Subjecting the human body to material ends*: The impermissibility of subjecting the human body to material ends may be deduced from the following two examples; Firstly, in the *fatwa*, it is stated that if a person, owing to hunger, finds himself on the verge of death, and is unable to find even the meat of a dead animal in order to save himself, and at that instant is offered human flesh, it would not be permissible for him to partake of it (Shafi 1967, 37).

Secondly, it is recorded in the *hadith* literature that Prophet Muhammad said that Allah denounces or curses the one who joins the hair of a woman to that of another so as to make her hair appear long — and that He also curses the woman with whose hair such hair is joined (*Sunan Abi Dawud. "Kitab al-Tarajjul." Hadith* no. 4168, 2:77). However, it is permissible for women to increase their locks by means of animal wool (Hamilton 1963, 270).

It may, therefore, be rightly inferred that since it is prohibited for Muslims to subject the human body to material ends and to make use of human hair, then by extension the use of parts of the human body, i.e. organs, will fall within the ambit of the prohibitions.

Al-Sukri makes a case against organ transplantation based on the following considerations:

*Sanctity of the human body*: On the basis of the *hadith*: "Breaking the bone of a dead person is equal in sinfulness and aggression to breaking it while a person is alive," the Muslim jurists make it a duty to re-inter human bones or remains if, for any reason, they are taken out of the graves. It is also equally obligatory to bury the limb that has been severed from a criminal, as well as human nails, hairs, etc. in honour of the sanctity of the human body (Al-Sukri 1989, 134).

*Prohibition of making use of forbidden things as medicines*: The following *hadith*, "Allah created the disease and also the cure, and for every disease He has provided a cure. So treat yourselves with medicines, but do not treat yourselves with prohibited things" (*Sunan Abi Dawud. "Kitab al-Jana'iz." Hadith* no. 3207, 2:212–3), renders utilizing human organs in treatment procedures impermissible by virtue of the fact that, as already cited, the Hanafi school regards making use of human bones in treatment as detestable (Al-Sukri 1989, 125).

*Safeguarding the honour of human life*: Abd al Rahman Ibn Uthman reports that a doctor came to the Prophet and asked him about the permissibility of making use of frogs in medicines and the Prophet forbade him from doing that. It can therefore be deduced that since this particular *hadith* censures the killing of frogs for the purpose of using them as medicines, it would therefore, be more prudent to safeguard the honour of human life by not allowing any human organs to be used in treatment procedures (Al-Sukri 1989, 136–7).

*Avoiding the doubtful act*: In a *Hadith*, Prophet Muhammad said, both legal and illegal things are obvious and in between, there are doubtful matters. So whoever forsakes those doubtful things lest he may commit a sin will definitely avoid what is clearly illegal; and whoever indulges in these doubtful things boldly, is likely to commit what is clearly illegal. Sins are Allah's *hima* (i.e. private pasture) and whoever pastures (his sheep) near it is likely to trespass in it at any moment (*Sahih Al-Bukhari. "Kitabal-Dhaba'i wa al-Sayd"*, 3:121–2).

In light of the above, therefore, utilizing human organs in transplantation procedures would be tantamount to indulging in the doubtful. Thus if one avoids resorting to organ transplantation, one would benefit in two ways. Firstly, if organ transplantation were to fall within the prohibited category, then one would have safeguarded oneself from trespassing the limits set by Allah. Secondly, if organ transplantation were to be within the permissible category then one would be rewarded for having avoided it lest it might be within the parameters of the forbidden (Al-Shukri 1989, 137). On the other hand, it must be emphasized that some Muslim scholars have also undoubtedly penned arguments in favour of organ transplantation, and others have issued positive religious decrees (*fatwa*) on this particular issue.

## Justifications for Organ Transplantation

Muslim jurists have justified organ transplantation on the basis of some Islamic juridical principles as follows:

*Public good (Al-maslahah)*: Both Sheikh Al-Bassam (1987, 13–22) and Sheikh Qabbani (1987, 27–32), concede that it is true that Islam forbids any act of aggression against human life as well as the human body after death. In other words then, if one were to take an organ out of the dead man's body so as to transplant it into another person, it could justifiably be argued to be tantamount to mutilation of the body and violation of the sanctity of the corpse. However, they argue that the Islamic legal system takes the interests of humans into consideration. For example, the juridical rules — necessity makes the unlawful permissible; when two interests conflict let the one which will bring greater benefit take precedence, and if forced to choose, choose the lesser of the two evils — are all founded on the principles of establishing what is in the general interest of public good and preventing what is against it. So, if the general gain outweighs the negative aspect of an action, it is allowed, but if the negative consequences of such an action outweigh the good then it is prohibited. In this context, for example, Ibn Qudamah (undated, 2:551) endorses the cutting of the belly of the dead pregnant woman in order to remove the fetus should any movement be detected within her uterus precisely because the right of the living supersedes consideration over that of the dead.

Likewise, Sheikh Darsh (1981, 3) points out that Islamic law would allow the cutting of the belly of the deceased who had swallowed a valuable diamond or a piece of gold in order that it may be returned to its rightful owner. The logical explanation for this is that if the valuable article had belonged to the deceased himself, then his/her heirs would be in a position to benefit from it. Hence, following the same line of argument, after a person has died it would be justified to retrieve the desired organ from that person's body for the purpose of its transplantation into that of another living person. This act would be regarded as a commendable gesture since the quality of life of the living would be enhanced as a result of this procedure.

Zahir (undated, 83), argues that Muslim scholars who advocate the permissibility of organ transplantation do not give outright approval for the practice. Zahir is of the view that the permissibility of organ transplantation should be hedged with certain restrictions such as: the transplantation is the only form (means) of treatment; the expected degree of success of this procedure is relatively high; the consent of the owner of the organ or of his heirs has been obtained; death must have been fully established by Muslim doctors of upright character before such a venture is undertaken; and the recipient has been informed of the operation and its implication.

*Altruism (Al-ithar)*: The Qur'an and *Sunna* exhort Muslims to co-operate with one another and to strengthen the bond of brotherhood among them. The Qur'an is imperative in this regard: "Help you one another in right-eousness and piety" (5:2), and from the *Sunna,* the following *hadith* may be cited: "The believers, in their love and sympathy for one another, are like a whole body; when one part of it is affected with pain the whole of it responds in terms of wakefulness and fever (*Sahih Al-Bukhari. "Kitab al-Adab,"* 3:12).

Thus in the light of the above teachings, a living person's gesture to donate one of his/her organs to a sibling or another person who may be in dire need of it should be viewed as an act of altruism; that is, some people sharing what they have for the benefit of others. Here again, Zahir (undated, 85), points out that the following restrictions should be applied: the consent of the donor must be obtained; the transplantation is the only form of treatment possible; there is no imminent danger to the life of the donor; the respective transplantation has been proven successful in the past. Moreover, Sheikh Jad al-Haqq (1999, 428) warns that a vital organ (like the heart) cannot be donated in view of the fact that this would result in the death of the donor. He explains that this prohibition has no excep-tion, whether or not the donor has given his/her permission. If that person gave permission for the transplantation of his/her vital organ into someone else's body it would be tantamount to suicide. On the other hand, if that person had not given any consent for his/her vital organ to be transplanted into someone else's body then the people who undertake doing that would be guilty of taking the life of that person without any justifiable cause. Sheikh Jad al-Haqq (1999, 429) explains that in view of the obligation to protect one's life, one cannot prefer the life of another over one's own except if it be for a higher objective like the protection of the Islamic faith (*din*) by giving one's life for the defence of Islam (*jihad*).

## The Prohibition of Sale of Organs in Islam

Insofar as the selling of human organs is concerned, Muslim scholars concur that such sale would be deemed *batil* (i.e. null and void) based on the following considerations. First, a person cannot trade in something of which he is not the owner (Al-Muslimun 1985, 85). Second, a *hadith* states that: "Amongst those who would be held accountable on the Last Day is one who sold a freeman and ate up the proceeds" (*Sunan Ibn Majah*, "*Kitab al-Ruhun*." *Hadith* no. 4, 2:816). Third, such a practice could lead to abuse in that it could result in the organs of the poor being sold in the market like any other commodity (Shafi 1967, 22). Thus if one were to sell a "freeman," the buyer would have no right over him during his lifetime since the contract of sale was prohibited (*haram*) from the very outset. As for the body of a person, living or dead, it is generally accepted that it belongs to Allah alone. It therefore follows that no one, and not even one's progeny, has any right to sell, donate, or dispose of another person's body (organs included) except in the manner prescribed by Islam, that is, by proper burial of the deceased.

## Procurement of Organs from Non-Muslims

Zahir (undated, 87), points out that the permissibility for Muslims to receive the organs of non-Muslims is based on the following two conditions: first, no organs are available from Muslims and second, a Muslim's life would be in danger should the transplantation not be carried out.

In order to circumvent the problem of Muslims becoming recipients of non-Muslim organs, some contemporary Muslim jurists are of the opinion that a Muslim's gesture in donating any of his organs is to be categorized as a collective obligation which if fulfilled by the few, absolves the generality (*fard kifayah*) (Dar al-Ifta' *Fatwa*, 15).

## Islamic Juridical Resolutions on Organ Transplantation

Following are resolutions on different types of transplantation.

***Resolutions on autotransplantation***: The Council of the Islamic Juridical Academy of the Muslim World League, in Makkah, Saudi Arabia, at its eighth working session (1985/1405 AH) resolved that it is permissible within *Shari'a* to take a part of the human body and transplant it into the same body, as well as removing the skin or bone in order to graft it to some other part of that same body (Al-Bassam *et al.* 1987/1408 AH, 40).

The Council of the Islamic Juridical Academy of the Organisation of Islamic Conference, in Jeddah, Saudi Arabia, at its fourth working session

(1988/1408 AH) resolved that from the *Shari'a* point of view, an organ may be transplanted from one part of the body to another part of that same body provided it could be ascertained that the benefits accruing from this procedure would outweigh the harmful effects thereof. Furthermore, it resolved that it is also permissible for such a procedure to be undertaken for the purpose of replacing a lost organ, or reshaping it, or restoring its function, or correcting a defect, or removing a malformation which was the source of mental anguish or physical pain (OIC Islamic Fiqh Academy 1985–1989/1406–1409 AH, 52).

The Islamic Juridical Academy of India (1992), at its first Islamic Jurisprudence Seminar in Delhi, in March 1989, resolved that it is valid to replace a part of a person's body with another part from the same person on the ground of necessity.

***Resolutions on homotransplantation/allotransplantation***: The Council of the Islamic Juridical Academy of the Muslim World League, at its eighth working session in Mekkah (1985/1405 AH), resolved that it is permissible within *Shari'a* to remove an organ from one person and transplant it into another person's body in order to save the life of that person or to assist in stabilizing the normal functioning of the basic organs of that person. Likewise, the Academy pointed out that such a procedure in no way violates the dignity of the person from whose body the organ had been removed. Hence, the act of donating one's organ is to be viewed as a permissible and praiseworthy act as long as the following conditions are met:

(i) That the donor's life is not harmed in any way;
(ii) That the donor voluntarily donates his/her organ without any form of coercion;
(iii) That the procedure is the only medical means available to alleviate the plight of the patient; and
(iv) That the success rate of the procedures for removing and transplanting the organ is relatively high (Al-Bassam *et al.* 1987/1408 AH, 40).

The Islamic Juridical Academy of India, at its first Fiqh (Islamic Jurisprudence) Seminar in Delhi in March 1989, resolved that transplantation of human organs is permissible in a desperate and unavoidable situation where the patient's organ has stopped functioning and there is present danger that he/she would lose his/her life if the organ were not replaced. It is also permissible for a healthy person, based on the opinion of medical experts, to donate one of his/her kidneys to an ailing relative (Islamic Fiqh Academy of India 1992).

Insofar as corneal transplantation is concerned, the Council of the Islamic Juridical Academy of the Organisation of Islamic Conference, Jeddah, Saudi Arabia, at its fourth working session (1988/1408 AH) resolved that from the *Shari'a* point of view such a procedure is permissible (OIC Islamic Fiqh Academy 1988/1408 AH, 52).

***Resolution on heterotransplantation***: The Council of the Islamic Juridical Academy of the Muslim World League, in Makkah, at its eighth working session (1985/1405 AH) resolved that it is permissible within *Shari'a* to transplant the organ of an animal which has been slaughtered according to Islamic rites and/or that of other animals (not eatable according to Islamic *Shari'a*, i.e. pig) out of necessity (Al-Bassam *et al.* 1987/1408 AH, 40). This resolution on heterotransplantation was also ratified by the Islamic Juridical Academy of India (1992) at its first Islamic Jurisprudence Seminar in 1989 in Delhi.

From the above resolutions, it appears that there is consensus among the different Islamic juridical bodies that a Muslim, while living, may donate one of his organs, but not a vital one such as the heart. Equally, a Muslim may become the recipient of human or animal organs. This brings us to the following two questions: is it permissible for a Muslim to make a will, while still alive, stipulating his/her consent to donate an organ after death; and who may assent to the donation of the dead person's organ in the event that no such clause has been stipulated in the deceased's will.

## Inclusion of Organ Transplantation in a Will

Modern science has made it possible to harvest the organ of the deceased and to transplant it into the living for the purpose of improving the latter's quality of life. The question that arises here is whether it is permissible for a person to include organ donation in his/her will.

As no explicit text (*nass*) exists either in the Qur'an or in the *Sunna* on this question, differences of opinion prevail among Muslim scholars.

The Islamic Fiqh Academy of India (1992), during its Second Fiqh Seminar in December 1989 in New Delhi, resolved that if a person directed that after his death his organ should be used for the purpose of transplantation (in a testamentary disposition, as it is commonly known), it would not be considered as a will (*wasiyyah*) according to *Shari'a*.

The arguments that may have influenced the adoption of this negative resolution are based on: firstly, the concept that human organ is a trust (*amanah*) from the Creator; and secondly, the stance that human organs cannot be valued or assigned a price as human possessions.

*Human organs — a trust (amanah)*: As mentioned above, there are Muslim jurists who regard the human body (including its parts) as a trust (*amanah*). Therefore, since a human being does not own his body, he/she cannot make a gift of any part of his/her body either during his/her lifetime or after death. Thus to include organ donation in one's will would not be permissible since one cannot give away that which one does not legally own.

*Human organs — invaluable*: The deceased's estate is termed in Arabic as *mal mutaqawwam* (asset upon which a price can be set). Muslim jurists are of the opinion that a human being (including his organs) is *mal ghayr mutaqawwam* (not able to be valued, i.e. no price can be set for it) (Tanzil-ur-Rahman 1980, 2:330). Thus it logically follows that since no price can be set for a human organ, the stipulation for it to be donated after one's death, is null and void. However, the Council of the Islamic Juridical Academy of the Muslim World League, Makkah, at its eighth working session (1985/1405 AH), resolved that it is permissible in *Shari'a* to remove an organ from a dead person and transplant it into a living recipient, on the condition that the donor was sane (*mukallaf*) and had wished it so (Al-Bassam *et al.* 1987/1408 AH, 40).

Likewise, the Council of the Islamic Juridical Academy of the Organisation of Islamic Conference (OIC), during its fourth session held in Jeddah (1988), resolved that it is permissible from the *Shari'a* point of view to transplant an organ from the body of a dead person if it is essential to keep the beneficiary alive, or if it restores a basic function to his body, provided it has been authorized by the deceased or by his heirs after his death or with the permission of concerned authorities if the deceased has not been identified or has no heirs (OIC Islamic Fiqh Academy 1988/1408 AH, 52–3).

The above (positive) resolutions, we may safely assume, provide a valid theoretical basis for the inclusion of organ donation in one's will. The considerations that have played a major role in influencing the adoption of these positive resolutions for the inclusion of organ donation in one's will relate to what are termed as (a) altruism (*al-ithar*) and generosity towards humankind; and (b) the rule of necessity (*al-darurah*).

In the context of altruism, a living person's gesture in willing to donate his/her cornea, for example, after death has taken place should be viewed as an act of altruism. After all, through corneal transplant, the donor would in effect have made a noble contribution in restoring the sight of another fellow human being suffering from corneal blindness.

Tanzil-ur-Rahman (1980, 2:341), a former Chief Justice of Pakistan, is of the opinion that the inclusion of corneal donation, for example, in one's will may be held permissible on the basis of the rule of necessity. He explains that the rule of necessity is based upon the juridical principle of juristic preference (*al-istihsan*), that the needs of the living are given preference over those of the dead. Thus allowing the inclusion of organ donation in wills could be a positive step in resolving organ donation shortages worldwide. However, the Islamic Juridical Academy of India, as pointed out above, resolved that any direction outlined in the will pertaining to the donation of one's organs for transplantation would be invalid and should not be honoured (Islamic Fiqh Academy of India 1992). Tanzil-ur-Rahman (1980, 2:327) holds the view that once a person has included organ donation in his/her will, it will be valid and enforceable in *Shari'a*, subject to the following conditions:

(i) The donation (by will) is motivated purely for human good and is without any monetary or other remuneration;

(ii) The recipient's need is genuine, of the nature of extreme and dire necessity, with no alternative treatment available, and duly certified by two Muslim medical practitioners of integrity; and

(iii) The legator (donor) leaves behind no heir. If there is an heir, obtaining the heir's consent, after death, shall be necessary. If any one of the heirs (if there is more than one heir) does not consent to it, the term of will relating to organ donation shall not be executed.

Insofar as who would have the authority to assent to a donation of a dead person's organs in the event that no organ donation has been stipulated in the deceased's will, the Council of the Islamic Juridical Academy of the Organisation of Islamic Conference and Tanzil-ur-Rahman concur that the legal heirs could give the necessary assent for that.

## Conclusion

Insofar as brain death is concerned, Dr. Muhammad Sulayman al-Ashqar (1985, 408), an expert in the field of Islamic jurisprudence in Kuwait, argues that a brain dead person should be considered virtually dead and should be treated as dead, thus permitting disconnection of resuscitation equipment or the removal of organs for transplantation. In other words, he likens brain death to the attainment of "unstable life." Muslim jurists hold unstable life to be the stage right before the body becomes lifeless, i.e. the process of spirit or soul departure (Al-Wa'il 1985, 449–50). During this stage, the person has no eyesight, is unable to talk and cannot engage in voluntary motion. Abd Allah Muhammad Abd Allah (1985, 370) points out that scholars belonging to the *Shafi'i* school of Islamic jurisprudence are of the view that if a murderer has caused his victim to reach the stage of unstable life, which is also termed the stage of the slaughtered or slain, and then another criminal attacks the same victim, then only the first criminal will be punished for murder, while the second criminal will be chastised for violating the sanctity of the dead.

Furthermore, the question arises whether the physician's act in retrieving organs from the dead for transplantation purposes constitutes a violation of the sanctity of the dead. As mentioned earlier, the Council of the Islamic Juridical Academy of OIC (1988), states that it is allowed to transplant an organ from a dead person if certain conditions are met. It is noteworthy that the recommendation made at the conclusion of the Seminar on Human Life: Its Inception and End of Life as Viewed by Islam in Kuwait in 1985 categorically states: "*Fiqh* scholars are inclined to the view that when it is ascertained that a human being has reached the stage of brain death, he is considered to have withdrawn from life." However, on the issue of retrieving organs from brain dead patients, the following remarks made by Tabatabaei (2014, 70), need to be carefully considered and reflected upon: "Although the transplantation of organs from brain dead patients in order to save human life is a laudable goal, the ethical and religious principle of protecting life and the soul should remain overriding considerations."

As for transplantation of human organs, it was pointed out that Muslim scholars differ on this issue. Following the establishment of Islamic Fiqh Academies in various parts of the Muslim world, there is at present consensus that Muslims may opt for this procedure in order to improve the quality of life. The author of this chapter strongly endorses the stance that organ transplantation, like blood transfusion, is a form of treatment. Hence, Muslims should avail themselves of this form of treatment as long as there is no other alternative. Moreover, consenting to donate one's kidney to someone else who is in dire need of it ought to be viewed as an act of sharing motivated by the spirit of love, compassion, and sympathy for a fellow human being. Muslims and followers of other religions believe that a dead human body must be treated with utmost respect. The Islamic juridical principle takes into consideration the interest of man by maintaining that the right of the living supersedes that of the dead, Therefore, it does not consider cadaveric transplantation as mutilation. It is permissible for a Muslim to include organ donation in his will. Muslims believe that everything belongs to Allah. However, no one can deny that every person has been given partial ownership, if not full, over whatever he disposes. Therefore, incorporating organ donation in one's will for the purpose of saving or enhancing another's life can in no way be termed as breach of trust (*khiyanah fi al-amanah*). After all, this gesture is motivated by the intention (*niyyah*) to assist a person in need. Thus although such a stipulation in a will may not in effect conform to the strict dictates of the *Shari'a*, the author of this chapter is inclined to argue that it would at least be morally binding on the part of the heirs to execute such a direction.

## References

Abd al-Basit, Badr al-Mutawalli. 1989. The End of Human Life. In: *The Proceedings of the Seminar on Human Life: Its Inception and End as Viewed by Islam*. Kuwait: Islamic Organization for Medical Sciences.

Abd Allah, `Abd Allah Muhammad. 1989. The End of Human Life. In: *The Proceedings of the Seminar on Human Life: Its Inception and End of Life as Viewed by Islam*. Kuwait: Islamic Organization for Medical Sciences.

Abu Dawud, Sulayman Ibn al-As`ath al-Sijistani. Undated. *Sunan Abi Dawud*. Beirut: Dar Ihya' al-Sunnat al-Nabawiyyah. *"Kitab al-Jana'iz."* *Hadith* no. 3207, 2:212–3.

_____ *"Kitab al-Tarajjul"*. *Hadith* no. 4168, 2:77.

Al-`Amari, `Abd al-Qadir ibn Muhammad. 1989. The End of Human Life. In: *The Proceedings of the Seminar on Human Life: Its Inception and End of Life as Viewed by Islam*. Kuwait: Islamic Organization for Medical Sciences.

Al-Ashqar, Muhammad Sulayman. 1989. The End of Human Life. In: *The Proceedings of the Seminar on Human Life: Its Inception and End of Life as Viewed by Islam*. Kuwait: Islamic Organization for Medical Sciences.

Al-Bassam, `Abd Allah, `Abd al-Rahman. 1987/1408 AH. Zira`at al-A`da'al-Insaniyyah fi Jism al-Insan. [*Human Organ Trans-plantation*]. In: *Majallat al-Majma` al-Fiqhi*. Rabitat al-`Alam al-Islami.

Al-Bukhari, Muhammad Ibn Isma`il. Undated. *Sahih Al-Bukhari*. Cairo: Dar al-Sha`b. 3 vols.

Al-Wa'il, T. 1985. The Truth about Death and Life in the Qur'an and the Stipulations of Islamic Law. In: *The Proceedings of the Seminar on Human Life: Its Inception and End of Life as Viewed by Islam*. Kuwait: Islamic Organization for Medical Sciences.

Al-Ghazali, Abu Hamid Ibn Muhammad. Undated. [*Ihya' Ulum al-Din*]. *Revival of Religion's Sciences*. Cairo: Matba`at al-Istiqamah, 4:494.

Al-Mahdi, Mr. 1989. The End of Human Life. In: *The Proceedings of the Seminar on Human Life: Its Inception and End of Life as Viewed by Islam*. Kuwait: Islamic Organization for Medical Sciences, 315.

Ardughdu, M. S. 1989. The End of Human Life. In: *The Proceedings of the Seminar on Human Life: Its Inception and End of Life as Viewed by Islam*. Kuwait: Islamic Organization for Medical Sciences.

Al Salami, Muhammad al Mukhtar. 1989. When Does Life End? In: *The Proceedings of the Seminar on Human Life: Its Inception and End of Life as Viewed by Islam*. Kuwait: Islamic Organization for Medical Sciences.

Al-Sukri, `Abd al-Salam. 1989/1409 AH. *Naql wa Zira`at al A`da'al-Adamiyyah min Manzur al-Islam*. [*Islamic Perspectives on Human Organ Transplantation*]. Nicosia: Al-Dar al-Masriyyah li al-Nashr wa al-Tawzi`.

Awdah, `Abd al-Qadir. Undated. *Al-Tashri` al-Jina'i al-Islami Muqaranah bi al-Qanun al-Wada`i*. Cairo: Dar al-Turath al-`Arabi. 2 vols.

Barnard, C. N. 1987. Reflections on the First Heart Transplant. *South African Medical Journal* 72(11), xix–xx.

Crowe, S. and Cohen, E. 2006. *Organ Transplant Policies and Policy Reforms*. Available at: http://www.bioethics.gov/background/crowepaper.html.

Dar al-Ifta' Fatwa No. 15. Available at: http://www.daralifta.org/Foreign/default. aspx [last visited Dec 9, 2016].

Darsh, S. M. 1981. *Islamic Health Rules*. London: Taha Publishers.

*Da`wah-o-Irshad Wing of the Islamic Research Academy*. 1979/1400 AH. *Sermons of the Holy Prophet Muhammad*. Islamabad: Islamic Research Academy.

Ebrahim, A. F. M. E. 2001. *Organ Transplantation, Euthanasia, Cloning and Animal Experimentation*. Leicester: The Islamic Foundation.

Ebrahim, A. F. M. and Haffejee, A. A. 1989. *The Shari`ah and Organ Transplants*. Durban. Islamic Medical Association of South Africa.

Elkadi, Ahmad. 1989. The Heart and its Relation to Life — Introduction to the Discussion of When Life Ends. In: *The Proceedings of the Seminar on Human Life: Its Inception and End of Life as Viewed by Islam*. Kuwait: Islamic Organization for Medical Sciences, 348, 363.

Evans, M. 1993. Dying to Help: Moral Questions in Organ Procurement. In: Dickenson, D., Johnson, M. and Katz, J. 1993 or 2000? *Death, Dying and Bereavement*. London: Sage Publications Ltd.

Frenkel, S. Organ-Trafficking Laws in Key Countries. Available at: http://www. csmonitor.com/2004/0609/p12s02-wogi.html.

Häring, B. 1972. *Medical Ethics*. Slough: St Paul Publications, 132.

Ibn Majah, Abu `Abd Allah Muhammad Ibn Yazid. Undated. *Sunan Ibn Majah*. Beirut: Dar al-Ihya' al-Kutub al-`Arabiyyah. 2 vols.

Ibrahim, Ahmad Shawqi. 1989. The End of Human Life. In: *The Proceedings of the Seminar on Human Life: Its Inception and End of Life as Viewed by Islam*. Kuwait: Islamic Organization for Medical Sciences.

Islamic Fiqh Academy of India. 1992. Developing a Religious Law in Modern Times. *Religion and Law Review*, 1(1), 178.

Ibn Qudamah, Muhammad `Abd Allah Ahmad Muhammad. Undated. *Al-Mughni*. Cairo: Maktabat al-Jamhuriyyah al-`Arabiyyah. 9 vols.

Jad al-Haqq, `Ali Jad al-Haqq. 1994. *Buhuth wa Fatawa al-Islamiyahfi Qadaya Mu`asarah — Murunatuh waTatawwuruh*. Cairo: Matba`ah al-Azhariyyah. 2 vols.

Lamb, D. 1993. Organ Transplants. In: Dickenson, D., Johnson, M. and Katz, J. 1993. *Death, Dying and Bereavement*. London: Sage Publications Ltd.

Lyons, C. 1970. *Organ Transplants: The Moral Issues*. London. SMC Press Ltd., 50–52, 56.

Mason, J. K. and McCall Smith, R. A. 1999. *Law and Medical Ethics*. London: Butterworths.

Mazkur, K. *et al.* (eds.). 1989. Report on the Fifth Session. In: *The Proceedings of the Seminar on Human Life: Its Inception and End of Life as Viewed by Islam*. Kuwait: Islamic Organization for Medical Sciences.

Mongomery, J. 2003. *Health Care Law*. Oxford: Oxford University Press.

*Al-Muslimun* [Saudi Arabian newspaper]. 21–28 December 1985/9–15 Rabi` II 1406 AH.

Organisation of the Islamic Conference's Islamic Fiqh Academy. 1985–1989/1406-1409 AH. *Resolutions and Recommendations*. Jeddah: *Matabi` Sharikat Dar al-`Ilm li al-Tiba`ah wa al-Nashr*.

Qabbani, `Abd al-Rahman al-Rashid Rida. *"Zira`at al-A`da'al-Insaniyyah fi Jism al-Insan."* In: *Majallat al-Majma` al-Fiqhi*. Rabitat al-`Alam al-Islami.1408 AH/1987.

Qasmi, Mujahid al-Islam.Ramadan, Safar, Dhu al-Qa`dah. 1988/1409 AH. *Dimaghi Mawt wa Hayat ka Nazriyat aur us par Payda Hone Wale Fiqhi Sawalat*. In: *Bahth-o-Nazar*. [*Islamic Jurisprudential Questions about Different Viewpoints on Brain Death and Life*]. Delhi: Offset Press.

Shafi`, Mufti Muhammad. 1967. *Insani Ada'ki Paivandkari — Shari`at al-Islami-yyah ki Roshni main*. [*Perspectives of Islamic Shari'a on Human Organ Transplantation*]. Karachi: Dar al-Isha`at.

Smith, H. L.1970. *Ethics and the New Medicine*. Tennessee: Abingdon Press, 130.

Tabatabaei, S. M. Revisiting Brain Death: An Islamic Concept. In: Alireza Bagheri (ed.). *Biomedical Ethics in Iran: An Application of Islamic Bioethics*. 2014. Christchurch: Eubios Ethics Institute.

Tanzil-ur-Rahman. 1980. *A Code of Muslim Personal Law*. Karachi: Islamic Publishers.

Abu `Abd Allah Muhammad Ibn Yazid Ibn Majah, *Sunan Ibn Majah*. Beirut: Dar al-Ihya' al-Kutub al- `Arabiyyah.

Yasin, M. N. 1989. The End of Human Life in the Light of the Opinions of Muslim Scholars and Medical Findings. In: *The Proceedings of the Seminar on Human Life: Its Inception and End of Life as Viewed by Islam*. Kuwait: Islamic Organization for Medical Sciences.

Zahir, F. I. Undated. *Hiwar Ma`a Tabib Muslim.* [*Dialogue with Muslim Physician*]. Cairo: Al-Risalah.

Zhorne, J. E. 1985. Organ Transplants: How Far Dare We Go? *Plain Truth* 50(7), 10–4.

# CHAPTER SEVEN

# An Ethical Account of Human Embryonic Stem Cell Research in the Islamic World

## Hakan Ertin and Ilhan Ilkilic

### Summary

Rapid technological developments in human embryonic stem cell research hold promises of future new medical treatment for a range of currently incurable chronic diseases. At the same time, stem cell research using human embryos raises radically new, previously unimaginable, ethical issues which pose a dramatic challenge to humankind. By analyzing the discourses on these ethical issues, this chapter argues that the cultural values and religious convictions of all stakeholders involved play a decisive role in formulating ethical positions. In the Islamic world too, stem cell research using human embryos provokes new discussions about the moral status of the embryo according to Islamic ethical norms. This chapter describes the theological and philosophical criteria applied in this debate and discusses some ethical positions *vis-à-vis* embryonic stem cell research formulated in the Islamic world, including official regulations existing in some Muslim countries.

## Introduction

Public debates as well as academic discourse widely agree upon the assertion that rapid developments in biomedical research not only offer new diagnostic techniques and therapeutic interventions, but also raise ethical dilemmas hitherto unimaginable in the history of humankind. Among these issues are ethical questions arising from research using human embryonic stem cells. The way in which this debate is conducted is inexorably linked to specific local cultures and traditions, as we can see from the following critical analysis of the respective arguments. In an Islamic discussion, a broad range of arguments is developed when dealing with complex bioethical issues, based on the specific nature of Islamic legal and ethical deliberation processes, and also influenced by various social phenomena and political factors (Ilkilic 2005; 2006a). Central topics in this debate are the moral status of the embryo; possibilities for curing diseases and alleviating suffering; assessment of the value of modern biomedicine; and the problem of distributive justice in allocating scarce resources.

This paper starts with an outline of Muslims' understanding of the health and the moral status of the embryo according to the basic sources of Islam; then moving on to describing ethical positions and practical regulations applied in some Muslim countries with diverse traditions, forms of government, and social structure. While most of the existing literature in this field is primarily descriptive, this article examines not only the arguments and their historical circumstances, but also provides a critical reflection on the theoretical basis underlying commonly held positions. In our view, this reflection is of paramount importance in establishing an open, constructive dialogue between different cultures and academic disciplines.

## The Islamic Concept of "Human Beings" and Health

From the point of view of Islam, the human being occupies the highest place among God's creatures and is God's Vicegerent (*khalīfa*) on earth. According to the Qur'an, the most important source for Muslims, the human being was created in an ideal form and provided with many gifts from God (95:4; 32:9; 67:23; 82:7–8). Health ranks among God's most important gifts and is considered a great blessing. The understanding of health as God's gift is an immediate starting point for individuals' responsibility to guard their own health. Muslims are convinced that a person is not the actual owner of his or her body, but merely its beneficiary in this life, a fact that obliges them to go about life lawfully and responsibly. This responsibility for one's own health, derived from the understanding of the body's God-given nature, has specific implications for the Muslim with regard to, for instance, dietary and hygienic measures to ensure a healthy life, as well as medical interventions in case of illness (Sachedina 2009).

Because of this central meaning of health, some scholars tend to assess medical research directed towards discovering new treatments of diseases as a religious duty (*fard kifaya*) (Sachedina 2009; Athar 2008; Al-Aqeel 2009). Whether stem cell research falls into this realm of research depends on the categorical value of health according to the Islamic notion of human beings. The high esteem for health suggests that a healthy condition is desirable and is to be pursued through a worthy lifestyle, but its value is not absolute. Health in itself is not the source of ethical norms and value concepts, but is a gift from God, one among other gifts, and is to be balanced — in case of a conflict of benefits — by the Islamic code of norms and value concepts. As a consequence, one cannot value life only by *degrees of health* or *degrees of sickness* — moreover, one cannot judge a *life's worth* or the *worthlessness of life*.

## The Moral Status of the Embryo

In Islamic history, discussions about the moral status of the embryo were usually triggered by ethical and legal issues in family life, such as terminating a pregnancy or the regulation of conception, etc. Philosophical questions and discussions, going back to the Aristotelian or Galenic tradition (Musallam 1990), developed later than legal discussions and were not decisive for Islamic jurisprudence (Motzki 1991). While systematic debates on the dignity of the embryo arose only after the establishment of the canonical schools of law (*madhhabs*) in the 8th and 9th centuries, earlier legal judgments regarding the termination of pregnancy, i.e., its cause and related sanctions, are known to us and go back to the time the of the so-called "rightly guided caliphs" (632–661) (Khoury 1981).

The Qur'an, the holy book and the most important ethical source for Muslims, describes in a few places the development of the human in the mother's womb, speaking of the breathing-in of the soul. As the Qur'an reads, "Thus, He begins the creation of man out of clay; then He causes him to be begotten out of the essence of a humble fluid; and then He forms him in accordance with what he is meant to be, and breathes into him of His spirit: and [thus, O men] He endows you with hearing, and sight, and feelings as well as minds" (32:7–9). Another passage explains the human development in the mother's womb, his coming into the world, his dying after a certain life span, and also his rising again in the Other World, all being components of a continuum with different ontological qualities. "Verily We created man from a product of wet earth; then placed him as a drop (*nutfa*) (of seed) in a safe lodging; Then fashioned We the drop a clot (*'alaqa*), then fashioned We the clot a little lump, then fashioned We the little lump bones, then clothed the bones with flesh, and then produced it as another creation. So blessed be God, the best of Creators! Then lo! After that ye surely die. Then lo! On the Day of Resurrection ye are raised (again)" (23:12–6). The Qur'an itself does not give any concrete indication as to the exact point in time when the ensoulment occurs. However, we find in the *hadith* (the sayings of the Prophet Muhammad) the following indication: "Each one of you is collected as a sperm (*nutfa*) in the womb of his mother for 40 days, and then turns into a clot (*'alaqa*) for an equal period (of 40 days) and turns into a piece of flesh (*mudgha*) for a similar period (of 40 days) and then God sends an angel and orders him to write things, i.e., his provision, his age, and whether he will be of the wretched or the blessed (in the Hereafter). Then the soul is breathed into him" (*Sahih al-Bukhārī*). However, there are other *hadiths* describing the embryo as being endowed with a soul at other points in time, for example, on the 40th, 42nd, or 80th day of pregnancy (Canan 1999).

An analysis of the judicial and ethical literature in the Islamic tradition shows that ensoulment assumes a central value in the discourse about the moral status of an embryo or fetus. Unanimity does not prevail, however, among the Muslim jurists, neither about the day of the ensoulment nor about its ethical relevance. Therefore, the judgments of Islamic schools of thought on human-induced abortion differ widely from one another. An abortion before the 120th day of pregnancy is allowed by some schools of thought, either with or without the requirement of social and/or medical indications. Other scholars prohibit abortion after 40 days. In Islam, all schools of thought agree that termination is forbidden after ensoulment, that is, after the fourth month (i.e. 120th day of pregnancy). After this point, an abortion can only be legitimized if the life of the pregnant woman is in danger (Aksoy 2005; Beloucif 2000; Yeprem 2006a; 2007). According to these arguments, ensoulment gives the embryo an exceptional moral status, which is decisive for the ethical assessment of any medical intervention affecting the embryo.

Up to this point the moral implications of ensoulment for stem cell research have not been sufficiently discussed. The embryo's right to protection prior to ensoulment depends on the verdict about the nature of the change in status produced by the breathing-in of the soul: Given that biological life precedes ensoulment, to say that the embryo only becomes human after receiving the soul would create an assumption that this event brings about a categorical change in the nature of the embryo. Such an assumption suggests there are no strong arguments against the destruction of the pre-ensoulment embryo. From this point of view, stem cell research using human embryos would be ethically acceptable, provided the aims of this research are considered legitimate. If, on the other hand, ensoulment only effects a gradual change in the moral value of the embryo, it would be very hard to argue against the embryo's right to protection from the very beginning of its existence. We understand the theologico-ethical position developed by one of the most influential thinkers of the Islamic middle ages, Al-Ghazālī (d. 1111), in his main work *Ihyā' 'ulūm ad-dīn*, ("Revival of Religion's Sciences") to support the latter position. According to him, the embryo remains the same living being throughout gestation, albeit equipped with different characteristics and capacities according to its successive stages of development. Hence, he demands the protection of life from its inception in the maternal womb, irrespective of its physical development and the moment of ensoulment. He defines the killing of this life a "crime," the degree of which however increases with the growing age of the embryo or fetus. Thus, he argues for a gradual right of protection for the embryo; which is to say that the moral status of the embryo changes only gradually, not categorically over time (Al-Ghazālī 1917).

A survey of the classical literature regarding the moment of ensoulment shows that a clear majority of authors believes this event to occur on the 120th day of pregnancy. In our view, this trend is to be understood as rather pragmatic: in order to pursue an abortion in court, it is necessary first to establish the pregnancy. Apart from some quite uncertain pregnancy tests in the Islamic middle ages, the only more or less unequivocal signs of pregnancy were the repeated lack of menstrual flow and the externally visible changes of the maternal body, either of which presupposes an extended period of observation (Weisser 1983). Also, it was problematic to ascertain if what "was expelled" with an abundant bleed was actually an embryo or some other kind of organic matter. Hence, even if jurists had decided to count the beginning of human life from actual conception, they would have lacked the equipment to detect a pregnancy at such an early stage. This line of argument could be considered the reason for the relatively long period of 120 days before an abortion is considered a crime, and also avoids unjust punishment of the defendants. A review of the debates of the 1960s and '70s regarding family planning, birth control, and abortion, shows a trend to move away from ensoulment and instead to focus on the Qur'anic prohibition to kill humans and their children (Abdul-Rauf 1977; Khoury 1981; Shaltūt 1971). Such a position regards the fertilized egg as worthy of protection right from the beginning. As we have seen, this argument is not based on theories of ensoulment, but rather on the Qur'anic prohibition to kill human life, which also includes a ban on killing children for fear of poverty. Representatives of this position also point out that birth control was brought up as a demand by women in the West whose interests it was meant to serve. In response, they refused to legitimize abortion and rather advocated for a struggle against poverty through a more equitable distribution of world resources, equality of opportunity and fight against corruption (Bowen 1997). Increased embryological knowledge and, most of all, the ability to visualize embryonic development in the womb have no doubt played an important role in the formation of a position towards protecting embryos. It remains an open question as how far these arguments, which have been formulated in a particular socio-political situation, can provide a stable basis for future debates.

## Ethical Assessment of Embryonic Stem Cell Research

The Islamic Code of Medical Ethics (1981), which was developed at the First International Conference on Islamic Medicine in Kuwait, in reference to the sacredness of human life in the womb, ascribes some degree of right of protection to the embryo. It states that only in case of medical emergency may a pregnancy be terminated: "The sanctity of life covers all its stages including intrauterine life of the embryo and fetus. This shall not be compromised by the doctor save for the absolute medical necessity recognized by Islamic jurisprudence."

Embryos used in stem cell research are inevitably destroyed in the course of research. However, as these embryos are potentially viable human beings equal to those implanted in the maternal womb, many scholars have equated stem cell research with abortion. Thus, it is not surprising that discussion about stem cell research center on the moment of ensoulment of the human embryo. As the scholar Isam Ghanem writes: "Embryo research is ... legal under Islamic jurisprudence provided the fetus is under 120 days old and provided both the mother and husband together consent to such research" (Ghanem 1991).

In western discourse, fertilized eggs prior to implantation are referred to as *pre-embryos* (Jones 1995). The First International Conference on Bioethics in Human Reproduction Research in the Muslim World in 1991 in Egypt took issue with this problematic concept and pleaded for research using only embryos left over after an *in vitro* fertilization (IVF) cycle: "The excess number of fertilized eggs (pre-embryo) can be preserved by cryo-preservation.... These pre-embryos can be used for research on methods of cryopreservation provided a free and informed consent is obtained from the couple." In this opinion the approval of the duly married couple, the exclusion of commercial interests and clear, scientifically verifiable, thera-peutic research goals are highlighted (Serour 1997). The Islamic Medical Association of North America (IMANA), whose members are Muslim physicians, accepts in its statement *Islamic Medical Ethics — The IMANA Perspective*, the use of spare embryos for research purposes: "3. Additional embryos produced by IVF between husband and wife can be discarded or given for genetic research, if not to be used by the same couple for a future attempt" (IMANA Ethics Committee 2005). These and other similar argu-ments are, however, only tenable if one accepts as a basis for decision-making those Islamic positions that allow abortion without a valid reason until the 40th or up to the 120th day. However, those positions which declare abortion as absolutely forbidden (*haram*) — so long as a pregnancy does not endanger the life of the mother — categorically demand the rejection of research on embryonic stem cells. It seems difficult to judge this position, which allows the killing of embryos only if valid reasons are established. Supporters of this position must decide if research on embryos is justified by the possibility of finding new forms of therapy for certain diseases. Such a justification is not easy to maintain if one considers classical arguments that reflect familial and social mores.

## Embryonic Stem Cell Research in Selected Muslim Countries

After discussing the criteria for determining the moral status of the embryo as well as theological and philosophical arguments concerning human embryonic stem cell research, we will now discuss positions on and regulation of stem cell research in selected Muslim countries.

**Iran:** In *Shi'a* Iran, religious authority, represented by the Grand Ayatollahs, has the highest religious power in the country. This is in contrast to the many other Muslim states' religious cadres, when it comes to creating legislations. It is important to note that Iran is not a secular state, therefore the assessment and practice in any field are based on the opinions of the religious authority. For instance, it provides clear and direct information about Islamic approaches to stem cell research, at least from as a *Shi'ite* perspective. Moreover, the country's religious constitution facilitates and speeds up the decision-making process. Even in cases where there exists no legal regulation on a certain subject, the religious authorities' stance can open the way for research. Another reason for Iran's dynamism in its decision-making mechanism is linked to the state's desire to increase its weight in the global political arena. All of these factors result in dynamic debates on ethics, reflected by the large number of articles by Iranian researchers published in international journals, not matched in quantity by those from other Muslim states (Saniei 2008). Iran occupies a significant position in the Muslim world in comparison with other Islamic states when it comes to taking decisions on medical practices and opening new approaches in ethical debates from a religious perspective. On the kidney transplantation issue, for instance, Iran is one of the few states in the world that has been able to solve the donor problem almost entirely: Previous long waiting lists for transplantation have been eliminated through a distinctive method applied since 1997, based on compensated kidney donation (Bagheri 2006). Similarly, Iran is also prominent among other Muslim countries with its remarkable progress and interest particularly in stem cell research.

One of the main reasons behind Iran's scientific motivation for stem cell research is the political and religious authorities' general support for science and technology in order to increase the global power and prestige of their country (Saniei 2008). In 2002, Grand Ayatollah Ali Khamenei issued a stem cell *fatwa* declaring experimentation with human embryonic stem cells consistent with *Shi'ite* Islam, thus legitimizing stem cell research in Iran (Schienberg 2009). From the *Shi'ite* perspective, using human embryos in stem cell research or for therapeutic cloning is permissible on condition that the embryonic stem cells are obtained in the "pre-ensoulment" stage of fetal development (Gheisari 2012). This support from the religious and political authorities through such positive decrees encouraged and intensified stem cell research in Iran, which has since been conducted successfully by the country's leading research institutions such as the Royan Institute. Iran is one of the first Muslim states in the group of countries, including Sweden, the UK, Japan, South Korea, and Singapore, to produce embryonic stem cells (Saniei 2008; 2012). In March 2003, the official Iranian press agency (IRNA) announced that the country was among the top 10 countries in the world that are capable of producing, cultivating, and freezing human embryonic stem cells (Jafarzadeh 2009). The need for oversight of officially supported stem cell research accordingly emerged and led to the creation of joint guidelines of the Iranian Ministry of Health and Tehran University of Medical Sciences, *Ethical Guidelines for Gamete and Embryo Research*, in 2005, to regulate and determine the specific circumstances for the use of human embryos in stem cell research and therapy. According to the main principles reflected in the guidelines, consisting of 22 articles, human dignity and rights such as privacy and confidentiality should be respected; participation in research should be informed and voluntary; and the benefits and harm caused by the research should be carefully taken into consideration. The guidelines prohibit the production of hybrids by using human and animal germ cells and of human embryos made specifically for research purposes and eugenics applications. Only surplus IVF embryos under 14 days of age can be used for research that includes destruction of the embryo (Saniei 2008; Gheisari 2012).

The Royan Institute for Reproductive Medicine in Iran was established in 1991 as a clinic to treat infertility. In 1998 the Iranian Ministry of Health approved it as the sole research institute to focus on cell research and undertake stem cell studies and therapy in the 2000s (Gheisari 2012). In 2004, the Royan Institute established a human embryonic stem cell line from an inner cell mass of a human blastocyst (Baharvand 2004). In 2006, the institute created Royana, the first cloned sheep in Iran, and in 2008, Hana, the first cloned goat in Iran and the fifth in the world (Gheisari 2012). Today, the Royan Institute has an extensive scope of research, including studies on stem cell biology and technology, reproductive bio-medicine, and animal biotechnology (Royan 2015). In addition to the Royan Institute, the Iranian Molecular Medicine Network (a network comprising more than 30 individual research institutes across the country) and the Shaheed Beheshti University of Medical Sciences are among Iran's other institutions working on regenerative medicine (Saniei 2012).

In 2009, the Iranian Council for Stem Cell Research and Technology Development was founded in order to develop stem cell research policies, to fund relevant studies conducted by scientists and students from universities and research organizations, and to organize workshops on stem cell research (Gheisari 2012; Miremadi 2013). After the first private attempts at cord blood banking in 2005, Iran's national cord blood bank was launched by the governmental Iran Blood Transfusion Organization (IBTO) in 2010. IBTO also founded the Iranian Stem Cell Donor Registry to help patients in need of hematopoietic stem cell transplants from peripheral or bone marrow stem cells donated by volunteers (Gheisari 2012; Stavropoulos-Giokas 2014; Cheraghali 2011). A study shows that in Iran, the public spending allocated to science by the government rose from 0.2 percent of GDP ($232 million) in 1990 to 0.6 percent of the GDP ($1.2 billion) in 2005. These funds not only enabled increased stem cell research, but also the non-pecuniary supports. According to the *Washington Times*, stem cell research in Iran has been allowed since 2002, which is much earlier than the permission granted in the United States by the Obama administration (*Washington Times* 2009).

**Egypt:** The importance of Egypt's contributions to stem cell research is highlighted by its remarkable influence on the entire *Sunni* Muslim world through the Islamic institutions located there, and its leading role in organizing conferences on an international level. For instance, the first International Conference on Bioethics in Human Reproduction Research in the Muslim World was held in Egypt in 1991. Three main religious authorities reside in Egypt; the Grand Mufti of the country, the Sheikh of Al-Azhar and the Committee of Fatwas of Al-Azhar University whose *fatwas* are said to be respected by most *Sunni* Muslim groups (Atighetchi 2007). Together, these three religious authorities exert a decisive influence on government action and in the formation of public opinion. Debates in the country mostly focus on human cloning, which is as strictly prohibited as in the rest of the Muslim world. In the words of the *mufti* of Egypt, "it contradicts Islamic legislation and is prohibited in all its forms because it contradicts with Islam" (Al-Sayyari 2005). However, looking at the conceptualization of the embryo in these debates, a possible approach might in the future be adopted to guide embryonic stem cell research. Authorities in Egypt tend to permit non-reproductive cloning to produce stem cells as mentioned in the *Recommendations of the Workshop on "Ethical Implications of ART for the Treatment of Infertility."* Along similar lines, Gamal Serour from Al-Azhar University considers non-reproductive cloning admissible if surplus embryos are used, but only within the first 14 days after conception. Yet, Hamdy al-Sayed, the president of the Egyptian Health Syndicate, adopts a stricter stance towards the subject, regarding the embryo as an early phase of human life, and therefore opposes its use in research (Atighetchi 2007).

**Tunisia:** In Tunisia, all experimentation on the embryo — which is regarded as a "potential person" — is rejected by *Opinion No. 1* issued by the Tunisian Medical Ethics Committee in 1997. Both reproductive and therapeutic cloning are included in this prohibition. Moreover, procuring an embryo for study, research, or experimentation is banned under Law No. 01–93 enacted in August 2001, which restricts embryonic stem cell research. Article No. 11 of the same law points out that gametes or embryos may be preserved only for therapeutic purposes, to help the couple procreate, whereas Art. No. 14 forbids gamete or embryo donation in assisted reproductive techniques (Tebourski 2004).

**Arab Peninsula:** Among the Gulf States, stem cell research activity in Saudi Arabia and Qatar should be highlighted. In Qatar, Weill Cornell Medical College is an active center in stem cell research. Saudi Arabia, where IVF is very commonly performed, aims to create the biotechnological capital of the Middle East on the site of Jeddah BioCity. However, researchers have to use legally aborted fetuses, while producing embryos for the purpose of research is prohibited. The admissibility of using surplus IVF embryos for research and therapeutic cloning is still a subject of debate (Atighetchi 2007). Similarly, a *fatwa* issued by the Fiqh Council of the Muslim World League (2003) allows the usage of stem cells for therapeutic or justified scientific research purposes if obtained from a legal source. Obtaining, cultivating, and using stem cells is permissible if derived from miscarried embryos or fetuses or from those that have been aborted for therapeutic reasons allowed by Islamic *Shari'a*, if parents agree. Moreover, leftover fertilized embryos from IVF that are donated by the parents are allowed to be used on the condition that they will not be implanted for non-permissible pregnancies. Moreover, using cells from fetuses that are aborted deliberately and without a medical reason permitted by *Shari'a* are not permissible.

**Turkey:** With more than 95 percent of its population officially being Muslim, Turkey is one of the few secular states in the Muslim world. Although Islamic approaches do not directly influence legislation or state institutions, they do play a significant role in defining people's attitudes towards controversial issues in the modern time. In accordance with its secular character, there is no centralized religious authority contributing in Turkey's policy-making process. However, the Department of Religious Affairs (*Diyanet İşleri Başkanlığı*) delivers opinions with regard to public debates (Ilkilic 2009).

In order to characterize the legal framework for stem cell research in Turkey, the Turkish Ministry of Health issued two circulars in 2005 and 2006, the latter including a guideline on stem cell research. In the first circular, the Ministry highlighted that various studies had been conducted on the potential use of stem cells in medicine in Turkey as well as throughout the world. Even though the results of these studies were promising for the treatment of many diseases, they also led to debates when embryonic stem cells were used. The Ministry also announced that it was in the process of creating legal regulations for embryonic stem cell research that still needed to be formulated in accordance with the requirements of modern science and public conscience. It stated that, though not banned, embryonic stem cell research should not be conducted until these regulations were finalized (Turkish Ministry of Health 2005).

In contrast to the moratorium on embryonic stem cell research announced in the 2005 circular, adult stem cell research was allowed. The second circular was issued in 2006, and a framework of procedures and regulations for adult stem cell research was formulated in the *Guidelines for Non-embryonic Stem Cell Research for Clinical Purposes* and included in its Appendix. This 2006 circular on stem cell studies emphasizes that stem cell transplantation has long been used as a treatment method, particularly for hematological and oncological diseases. The circular also recognizes that the use of stem cells for therapeutic purposes has come under scrutiny in recent years. Intensive research on therapeutic stem cell transplantation continues in Turkey and throughout the world. However, although it is considered a promising treatment method for some diseases, the number of patients who have had stem cell transplantation is very low and there is insufficient data on the success of the practice or the long term side effects. The circular also announced that, together with the *Guidelines for Non-embryonic Stem Cell Research for Clinical Purposes*, a Scientific Advisory Board of Stem Cell Transplantation was established in order to create the necessary infrastructure and oversight within research institutions to ensure the conduct of research in accordance with the requirements of modern science (Turkish Ministry of Health 2006). As noted from the circulars, the Turkish Ministry of Health differentiates between embryonic and adult stem cell research. Although the Ministry has urged no embryonic stem cell research until relevant legal regulations have been finalized, it has allowed adult stem cell research through the 2006 circular that includes the aforementioned guideline regulating adult stem cell research. Following the Ministry's approach, stem cell research in Turkey concentrates mostly on stem cells derived from adults.

Beyond these guidelines and circulars, the *Regulations on Clinical Trials of Drugs and Biological Products* should also be taken into consideration (Turkish Drug and Medical Device Institution 2014). The former *Regulations on Clinical Research*, which had been in force in Turkey since 2009, were redrafted in 2014 into the *Regulations on Clinical Trials of Drugs and Biological Products*; and this new version came into effect on June 25, 2014. According to Articles 1 and 2, this regulation addresses the principles of scientific research on humans; the protection of research participants' rights; and the establishment and mandate of the Clinical Research Advisory Board and the ethics committees. The law also regulates clinical research of medical, biological, and herbal drugs involving human subjects whether conducted by individual researchers or a corporate entity. In this regulation there are no particular sections specifically addressing stem cell research. The regulation requires that in the absence of relevant specifications, the following guidelines or regulations should be complied with: internationally (1) the *Convention for the Protection of Human Rights and Dignity of the Human Being with Regard to the Application of Biology and Medicine*; and nationally (2) the *Medical Deontology Regulations*; and (3) the *Regulations on Patients' Rights*. Accordingly, these three regulations will be discussed next with respect to stem cell research.

Stem cell research, which holds tremendous promise for the development of therapies to regenerate damaged organs and to cure a variety of diseases that conventional medicine has so far not been able to cure, can be evaluated in the light of Articles 10 and 11 of the *Medical Deontology Regulations* (1960), and Article 27 of the *Regulations on Patients' Rights*. Both regulations highlight the inability of conventional medical techniques to cure certain diseases and the necessity to conduct adequate animal experimentation before inventing new medical treatments. Article 11 of the *Medical Deontology Regulations* states: "When it has been proven by clinical or laboratory examination that the patient does not benefit from conventional medical techniques, a treatment method of which beneficial effects have been confirmed following adequate experimentation on animals can be implemented." Similarly, Article 27 of the *Regulations on Patients' Rights* (1998) states: "When it has been proven by clinical or laboratory examination that the patient does not benefit from conventional medical techniques, a different treatment modality instead of the conventional medical techniques can be used, provided that the beneficial effects of this method have been ascertained by adequate animal experimentation, and that the patient consents to it. In addition, if a non-established treatment modality instead of the conventional techniques is to be used, it must be likely that the new method will be beneficial for the patient and not cause less favorable results than those of the conventional methods." Therefore, the stem cell research can be considered as a new medical treatment method addressed by these articles.

The Council of Europe (CoE) Convention for the Protection of Human Rights and Dignity of the Human Being with Regard to the Application of Biology and Medicine, also known as the Oviedo Convention on Human Rights and Biomedicine (the Oviedo Convention for short), is the first international treaty in this field; and Turkey signed the convention in 2003. At this point, it is important to consider the legal status of international treaties in the Turkish legal system. Article 90 of the Turkish Constitution states that: "In case of conflict between international treaties, in the area of fundamental rights and freedoms that have been duly put into effect, with domestic laws due to differences in provisions on the same matter, the provision of the international treaties shall prevail." Therefore, international treaties signed by Turkey, including the Oviedo Convention, act as a source for medical law (Sert 2011).

Article 18 of the Oviedo Convention addresses stem cell research in particular. Article 18(1) requires that any embryo undergoing research should be provided due protection, stating: "Where the law allows research on embryos *in vitro*, it shall ensure adequate protection of the embryo." Article 18(2), moreover, states: "The creation of human embryos for research purposes is prohibited." The Oviedo Convention should be considered together with the Turkish Ministry of Health's *Legislation Concerning the Practices and Centers of Assisted Reproduction Treatment*, which is a comprehensive piece of legislation providing definitions and addressing practices of assisted reproduction treatment, detailing the prohibitions as well as all the requirements that clinics must fulfill to obtain a license to practice (Turkish Ministry of Health 2014; Gürtin 2012). According to Annex 17(3), "the storage, use, transfer, and sale of egg and sperm cells provided from the spouses to undergo assisted reproduction treatments and of the embryos produced from these cells for any purpose except those that have been defined in this legislation are prohibited."

As for excess embryos originating from the procedures involved in assisted reproduction, using those embryos would not mean a violation of Article 18(2) of the Oviedo Convention unless they are intentionally produced for research purposes (Karakaya 2013). Article 20(5) of the *Legislation Concerning the Practices and Centers of Assisted Reproduction Treatment* states that excess embryos can be frozen and stored with the consent of the both spouses. In case the duration of storage exceeds one year, the spouses must re-apply every year with a signed petition stating that their demand for the preservation of the embryo is still valid. Upon the request of the couple, or in case either of the spouses dies or they obtain a divorce, or when the fixed period of storage has ended, the embryos are destroyed, the process of destruction being recorded by a committee to be established within the Directorate.

In addition, according to Article 20(6), "embryos shall be stored no longer than five years. A storage period of more than five years is only possible with the permission of the Ministry of Health."

In Turkey, both the number of stem cell transplants and the number of stem cell research centers and laboratories has rapidly increased during recent years. As of 2012, the total number of adult stem cell transplants was 2,032 cases in adults and 560 cases in children. There are currently 20 pediatric stem cell transplant centers in Turkey, where the first transplant center was established in 1989. As of March 2014, stem cell research in Turkey is performed at one dedicated Stem Cell Institute in Ankara University; four research and development centers; four Good Manufacturing Practices laboratories authorized by the Ministry of Health. There are five similar laboratories waiting to be authorized by the Ministry of Health (Can 2014).

From a religious perspective, the Religious High Council under the Directorate of Religious Affairs, the senior official religious authority in Turkey, issued a series of opinions with regard to IVF, stem cells, and rights of the fetus. Their report particularly emphasized that the number of embryos produced during IVF treatment should remain at a minimum level, as the destruction of surplus embryos raises serious doubts from the religious point of view, given that embryos can be regarded as human beings and as such must be respected in the first instance. If because of medical necessities or technical (im)possibilities more embryos are produced than the number of babies intended to be gestated, the number of additional embryos should be kept to a minimum and surplus embryos should be reserved for stem cell research rather than be destroyed. Stem cell production is thus allowed, provided the embryos are obtained in this way (Yeprem 2006b). On the other hand, the use of embryos in early stages is considered permissible under certain circumstances: where it is not possible to obtain stem cells with the characteristics of embryonic stem cells from differentiated adult cells and there is no other possible method of treatment, blastocysts left over from IVF can be used for therapeutic purposes on the condition that all necessary measures are taken against their commercial use and any sort of misuse (Yeprem 2006b; RHCDRA undated).

For Hayrettin Karaman, a prominent scholar of Islamic law in Turkey, laboratory-produced embryos cannot be considered as human beings unless they are implanted in the uterus, and thus their destruction can be seen as permissible. Surplus human embryos should be used for stem cell research purposes, however, and not for cloning. Although positive attitudes towards scientific research and development seem to prevail in Islamic countries in general, this does not mean that there are no significant differences between individual Islamic scholars. Karaman maintains that laboratory-produced embryos cannot be considered human beings, and that it is permissible to use embryos produced from the sperm and ova of unmarried men and women if their purpose is research or tissue production. Moreover, he evaluates this situation as being similar to that of obtaining tissues from an unknown third person. Karaman has no objection to the destruction of lefto-ver embryos since they cannot be regarded as a human being (Karaman 2005). In contrast, others consider laboratory production of embryos as improper, as evidenced by a report titled *Evaluating the Highly Debated New Implementations of Today's Medicine such as IVF and Stem Cell with Regard to the Religion of Islam* issued by the Department of Religious Affairs in January 2006 which states that a human should be respected as an individual "from the beginning;" therefore, only leftover embryos from IVF should be used in stem cell research (RHCDRA undated).

## Debates on Embryonic Stem Cell Research: Some Reflections

In the existing academic literature, the positions and arguments about stem cell research are mostly on a descriptive level. We argue that straight-forward and comprehensive reflection is needed to reach an adequate understanding of these positions.

## Moral assessment of the utility of stem cell research

Currently, hope for healing incurable diseases is one of the crucial moral premises for a supportive assessment of human embryonic stem cell research (Siddiqi 2002; Larijani 2004; Rizvi 2004; Hathout 2006; Ilkilic 2008; Saniei 2008; Sachedina 2009; Al-Aqeel 2009). There is an expectation that in the foreseeable future this research activity will lead to concrete therapeutic options for numerous diseases. Such a result has been rightly considered useful, both from the individual perspective and for the public interest (*maslaha*) (Khadduri 1991). However, from the viewpoint of medical experts, such an enthusiastic anticipation seems to be disingenuous. It cannot be denied that research is still at the basic stage, which is to say that innovative, validated stem cell therapies are not expected any time soon. The discussion does not yet reach the required level for a sophisticated analysis of the opportunities and limitations of stem cell research; leaving the debate within Islam with severe deficiencies, especially with regard to technical details. It can be claimed that stem cell research — even where it does not immediately lead to the cure of specific diseases — may contribute significantly towards a better understanding of physiological and pathophysiological processes at the cellular level. From the perspective of Islamic ethics, the utility of this increase in knowledge could in any case be valued positively. This kind of assessment to support these kinds of research is understandable, yet it requires more careful analysis of the whole situation.

As it stands, the potential goods and outcomes weighed against each other are changing in their nature: no longer is there a balance to be struck between "cure of disease versus killing of the embryo," but now the issue is between "increase of knowledge versus killing of the embryo" — a distinction which is sorely missed in the contemporary debate.

## Moral assessment of embryo's ensoulment

In many positions argued today, the normative determination of the ensoulment of the embryo turns out to be the pivotal point for the moral assessment of stem cell research. First of all, in the classical method of religious adjudication it needs to be clarified that to what degree the ensoulment of the embryo offers a sufficient moral basis for the absolute protection of the embryo? Explicit statements about a normative nexus between an embryo's ensoulment and its entitlement to protection are not to be found in either the verses of the Qur'an or the traditions of the Prophet (*Sunna*). It is unfortunate to see that this problem has not been specifically addressed in the discussion of this issue. Instead, we need to ask how such an open-ended question of stem cell can be assessed through the classical means of Islamic *Shari'a*. However, in the absence of explicit debates about these questions in the Islamic *Shari'a*, it is not possible to integrate their results into the stem cell research debates. The complexity of this situation does however indicate that further studies in this area proposing appropriate approaches are required for further debate.

## Normative implications of ensoulment

In the inner-Islamic discussion, there is no doubt that the question of ensoulment of the embryo plays a normative role in the moral assessment of stem cell research. At this point, it is worth asking from where this normative role can and does arise.

When addressing this question, it seems to be important to establish if we can find another comparable situation in a different stage of life. As an analogy, we can think about the end of life given that Islam defines death as the separation of the soul from the body, after which the human body is considered a corpse with a lower moral status than that of a living person's body. Nevertheless, the physical integrity of the dead body is of great importance — for instance, a cadaver must not be opened surgically unless there is an important reason. However, the moral status of a cadaver is not identical to that of a living human body. Now we can ask if the status of an embryo or fetus before ensoulment at the beginning of life can be analyzed in a morally equivalent way. In the case of a dead person, we are confronted with a lifeless body where no organs are working and the body no longer functions as a biologically integrated organism. By contrast, an embryo, or rather fetus, of 120 days' gestational age has a beating heart and, under the conditions of the existence in the womb, a functioning lung and a renal–urinary system. Even though this living being is not yet viable outside the mother's womb, it needs to be considered as an integrated, functioning, living organism. What is more, this body has the potential to develop into a human person. In this respect, in the context of biology, there is a crucial, categorical difference between the two states. It thus seems problematic to treat the fetus and the dead body as morally equivalent based on the absence of a soul.

Another relevant question in the moral assessment of research involving the destruction of embryos is to analyze whether the notion of ensoulment is a workable normative concept. The Qur'anic verses and Prophetic *hadiths* mentioning ensoulment are describing development *in utero* as an expression of divine omnipotence. In this respect, the description of the concomitantly mentioned ensoulment of the embryo does not seem to serve as an applicable normative concept. This argument needs to be followed up by experts in Qur'anic exegesis and *hadith* scholars, which is beyond the scope of this paper. It should be noted that a comprehensive reflective debate is needed, given that such a discussion has not yet been held among Muslim scholars.

## Plurality of opinions and the limits of casuistic arguments

A number of reasons accounts for the plurality of opinions in the Islamic debate regarding research using human embryonic stem cells. An important aspect is the Islamic method of legal deliberation, which is based on casuistry, i.e., analyzing a current action or misdeed on the basis of legal precedents. To this day, jurists argue on the basis of analogies harking back to classical arguments drawn from earlier Islamic intellectual history. Applying different methods or divergent assessments of an ethical norm inevitably leads to pluralism, which can be observed between the different schools of law throughout the Islamic world. What is more, there is no hierarchy of legal experts, of the type that exists, for example, in the Roman Catholic Church. This makes it impossible to declare one particular decision as the will of God. This pluralism, a matter of Muslim contentment, offers a wider realm for decisions of conscience, yet at the same time, it may pose a great challenge to of the consistency of decision-making.

It should be noted that the method of casuistry reaches its limits when it comes to the question of killing embryos for the purpose of research. In the traditional assessment, conflicts concerning the mother, family, or society are directly analyzed and balanced against other harms and benefits. It seems clear that this way of reaching a verdict cannot easily be applied as a foundation for decisions regarding research using human embryos, given the incommensurable quality of the goods to be balanced.

## Perceptions of modern science and technology

While rarely reflected in academic debates, the assessment of stem cell research is greatly influenced by the understanding of modern medicine and western technology. Different perceptions of modern science and its application in daily life play an essential — if not decisive — role in the ethical assessment of stem cell research using human embryos. In this discourse, two predominant positions are noticeable. The first position is based on an absolutely positive attitude to the contributions of scientific research and technological developments in every area of life. According to this position, modern science and research and their applications are ethically neutral, objective, and value-free. There are no connections between culture and technology. The advocates of this position argue that substantially there is no morally good or bad research and technology. Therefore, research and technology need to be ethically assessed only according to their goals and applications (Ilkilic 2006b; Hoodbhoy 1991).

The second position in this discourse, held especially by Muslim intellectuals and philosophers, emphasizes the inseparable character of culture from scientific research and technologies. They argue that owing to the secular character of scientific developments in the 19th and 20th centuries, Muslims should maintain a critical attitude towards western science. The main point is whether the concept of humankind on which scientific research is based is compatible with that upheld in Islamic belief (Ilkilic 2006b; Açıkgenç 1996; Anees 1989). If not, Muslims should be critical with regard to such scientific research and developments in the West, and stem cell research with human embryos would fall into this category as well.

## Just allocation of medical resources

Stem cell research requires know-how, financial resources, and scientific infrastructure. Only a few Muslim countries can match these conditions.

Due to a lack of such resources, stem cell research is not a "hot topic" for most Muslim countries. Yet, there is another eminent issue in the ethical assessment of stem cell research needing attention, namely the justification of allocating scarce resources within the healthcare system. In most Muslim countries, even basic healthcare is lacking, and these countries do not have enough resources to establish an accessible basic medical care system. To many experts, the diversion of existing resources into basic research in such circumstances does not seem ethically justifiable. They argue that an investment into long-term medical research instead of urgent healthcare programs cannot be acceptable, especially where public interest (*maslaha*) is considered.

## Conclusions

Bioethicist LeRoy Walters from Georgetown University distinguishes six possible policy options regarding human embryo and human embryonic stem cell research:

> Option 1: No human embryo research is permitted, and no explicit permission is given to perform research on existing human embryonic stem cells; Option 2: Research is permitted only on existing human embryonic stem cell lines, not on human embryos; Option 3: Research is permitted only on remaining embryos no longer needed for reproduction; Option 4: Research is permitted both on remaining embryos (see Option 3) and on embryos created specifically for research purposes through *in vitro* fertilization (IVF); Option 5: Research is permitted both on remaining embryos (see Option 3) and on embryos created specifically for research purposes through somatic cell nuclear transfer into human eggs or zygotes; and finally Option 6: Research is permitted both on remaining embryos (see Option 3) and on embryos created specifically for research purposes through the transfer of human somatic cell nuclei into nonhuman animal eggs, for example, rabbit eggs (Walters 2004).

According to the ethical arguments and criteria discussed in the Islamic world we have laid out above, it seems possible to say that option 3 is a widely accepted position among the majority of Muslim scholars and most of the Muslim countries, and options 4, 5, and 6 are rejected.

However, these arguments and positions lead us to the following conclusions: First, the dominant position in the Muslim world is to support this kind of research. Second, the ethical assessment of stem cell research using human embryos in the Islamic world is varied. The third is that the discourse about stem cell research involves essential problems because of the methods of argument used and the complex character of stem cell research. Finally, a better ethical assessment of stem cell research needs a holistic approach, and interdisciplinary and international research.

## References

Abdul-Rauf, M. 1977. *The Islamic View of Women and the Family.* New York: Robert Speller and Sons.

Açıkgenç, A. 1996. *Islamic Science: Towards a Definition.* Kuala Lumpur: ISTAC.

Aksoy, S. 2005. Making Regulations and Drawing up Legislation in Islamic Countries Under Conditions of Uncertainty, with Special Reference to Embryonic Stem Cell Research. *Journal of Medical Ethics*, 31(7), 399–403.

Anees, M. A. *Islam and Biological Futures: Ethics, Gender, and Technology.* London: Mansell, 1989.

Al-Aqeel, A. I. 2009. Human Cloning, Stem Cell Research: An Islamic Perspective. *Saudi Medical Journal*, 30(12), 1507–14.

Al-Bukhārī, Muhammad ibn Ismail. 1985. *The Translation of the Meanings of Sahih al-Bukhari: Arabic–English, Volume 8.* Trans. Khan, M. M. Beirut: Darussalam.

Al-Ghazālī, Abū Ḥāmid Muḥammad ibn Muḥammad. 1917. In: *Islamische Ethik, nach den Originalquellen übersetzt und erläutert, h. 2: Von der Ehe: das 12. Buch von al-Gazalis Hauptwerk* [Ihyā' 'ulūm ad-dīn]. [Islamic Ethics: According to Original Translated Sources. Based on Al-Gazali's book: *Revival of Religion's Sciences*].

Al-Sayyari, R. A. 2005. Ethical Aspects of Stem Cells Research. *Saudi Journal of Kidney Diseases*, 16(4), 606–11.

Athar, S. 2008. Enhancement Technologies and the Person: An Islamic View. *Journal of Law, Medicine & Ethics*, 36(1), 59–64.

Atighetchi, D. 2007. *Islamic Bioethics: Problems and Perspectives.* Dordrecht: Springer.

Bagheri, A. 2006. Compensated Kidney Donation: An Ethical Review of the Iranian Model. *Kennedy Institute of Ethics Journal,* 16(3), 269–82.

Baharvand, H., Ashtiani, S. K., Valojerdi, M. R., *et al.* 2004. Establishment and *In Vitro* Differentiation of a New Embryonic Stem Cell Line from Human Blastocyst. *Differentiation,* 72(5), 224–9.

Beloucif, S. 2000. The Muslim's Perspective Related to Stem Cell Research. In: European Group on Ethics in Science and New Technologies (EGE). *Adoption of an Opinion on Ethical Aspects of Human Stem Cell Research and Use.* Brussels: EGE, 119–23.

Bowen, D. L. 1997. Abortion, Islam, and the 1994 Cairo Population Conference. *International Journal of Middle East Studies,* 29(1), 161–84.

Can, A. and Demirer, T. (eds.). 2014. *Ulusal Kök Hücre Politikaları Çalıştayı Raporu. [Report of the National Stem Cell Policies Workshop].* Ankara: TÜBA, 32–3.

Canan, I. 1999. *Kütüb-i Sitte Muhtasarı Tercüme ve Şerhi [Translation and Commentary on Six Books Compendium]. Volume* 14(13). Ankara: Akçağ.

Cheraghali, A. M., Amini-Kafiabad, S., Amirizadeh, N., *et al.* 2011. Iran National Blood Transfusion Policy: Goals, Objectives and Milestones for 2011–2015. *Iranian Journal of Blood and Cancer,* 3(2), 35–42.

Ghanem, I. 1991. Embryo Research: An Islamic Response. *Medicine, Science and the Law,* 32(1), 14.

Gheisari, Y., Baharvand, H., Nayernia, K. and Vasei, M. 2012. Stem Cell and Tissue Engineering Research in the Islamic Republic of Iran. *Stem Cell Reviews and Reports,* 8(3), 629–39.

Gürtin, Z. B. 2012. Assisted Reproduction in Secular Turkey: Regulation, Rhetoric, and the Role of Religion. In: Inhorn, M. C. and Tremayne, S. (eds.). *Islam and Assisted Reproductive Technologies: Sunni and Shia Perspectives.* New York: Berghahn Books, 291.

Hathout, H. 2006. An Islamic Perspective on Human Genetic and Reproductive Technologies. *Eastern Mediterranean Health Journal,* 12(Supp. 2), 22–8.

Hoodbhoy, P. 1991. *Islam and Science: Religious Orthodoxy and the Battle for Rationality: Coexistence and Conflict.* London: Zed Books.

*Islamic Code of Medical Ethics: The Kuwait Document.* 1981. Kuwait: International Organization of Islamic Medicine.

Ilkilic, I. 2005. New Bioethical Problems as Challenge for Muslims and Health Literacy in a Value-Pluralistic Society. *Chennai Journal of Intercultural Philosophy*, 7, 72–92.

Ilkilic, I. 2006a. Human Cloning as a Challenge to Traditional Health Cultures. In: Roetz, H. (ed.). *Cross-Cultural Issues in Bioethics: The Example of Human Cloning*. Amsterdam: Rodopi, 409–23.

Ilkilic, I. 2006b. Modernisierung und Verwestlichung-Diskussionen und bioethische Fragen am Beispiel der innerislamischen Diskursen. [*Modernization and Westernization: Bioethical Questions, Using the Example of the inner-Islamic Discourses*]. In: Eich, T. and Hoffmann, T. S. (eds.). *Kulturübergreifende Bioethik, zwischen globaler Herausforderung und regionaler Perspektive.* [*Inter-cultural Bioethics, Between Global Challenges and Regional Perspectives*]. Freiburg: Verlag Karl Alber, 142–51.

Ilkilic, I. 2008. Stammzellforschung: Die innerislamische Diskussionslage [*Stem Cell Research: The Inner-Islamic Discussion*]. In: Körtner, U. H. J. and Kopetzki, C. (eds.). *Stammzellforschung: Ethische und rechtliche Aspekte* New York: Springer, 222–32.

Ilkilic, I. and Takim, A. 2009. Bioethik am Beispiel der Stammzelldebatte in der Türkei. In: Joerden, J. C., Moos, T. and Wewetzer, C. (eds.). *Stammzellforschung in Europa:religiöse, ethische und rechtliche Probleme*. Frankfurt am Main: Peter Lang, 183–97.

IMANA Ethics Committee 2005. Islamic Medical Ethics: The IMANA Perspective. *Journal of Islamic Medical Association*, 37(1), 38.

Jones, D. G. and Telfer, B. 1995. Before I Was an Embryo, I Was a Pre-Embryo: Or Was I? *Bioethics*, 9, 32–49.

Karakaya, A. 2013. *Stem Cell Research and Ethics/Ethical Issues in Studies of Stem Cells Derived from Human Embryos*. Master's thesis. Istanbul, 49–50.

Karaman, H. 2005. *Kök hücre*. Available at www.hayrettinkaraman.net/yazi/laikduzen/4/0109.htm (in Turkish). Accessed 22 December 2009.

Khadduri, M. 1991. Maslaha. [*Interest*]. In: *The Encyclopaedia of Islam, Volume 6.* 2nd ed. Leiden: Brill, 738–40.

Khoury, A. T. 1981. Abtreibung im Islam. [*Abortion in Islam*] CIBEDO-Dokumentation, Nr.11, 8–11.

Larijani, B. and Zahedi, F. 2004. Islamic Perspective on Human Cloning and Stem Cell Research. *Transplantation Proceedings*, 36(10), 3188–9.

Medical Deontology Regulations. In: *Official Gazette*, 19 February 1960, no. 10436. Available at: www.resmigazete.gov.tr/arsiv/10436.pdf (in Turkish). [Accessed 2 May 2016].

Miremadi, T. 2013. Biotechnology in Iran: A Study of the Structure and Functions of the Technology Innovation System. In: Soofi, A. S. and Ghazinoory, S. (eds.). *Science and Innovations in Iran: Development, Progress, and Challenges*. New York: Palgrave Macmillan, 139–59.

Motzki, H. 1991. *Die Anfänge der islamischen Jurisprudenz: ihre Entwicklung in Mekka bis zur Mitte des 2./8. Jahrhunderts*. [*The Beginnings of Islamic Jurisprudence: Its Development in Mecca Until the Middle of the 2nd/8th Century*.] Stuttgart: Steiner.

Musallam, B. 1990. The Human Embryo in Arabic Scientific and Religious Thought. In: Dunstan, G. R. (ed.). *The Human Embryo, Aristotle and the Arabic and European Traditions*. Exeter: University of Exeter Press, 32–46.

Muslim Word League. 2003. *Fatwa number 3: Regarding stem cells*. Islamic Jurisprudence Council Conference, December 13–7, 2003, Mekka, Saudi Arabia. Available at: www.themwl.org/Fatwa/default.aspx?d=1&cidi=152&l=AR&cid=12 (in Arabic). [Accessed 22 December 2009].

Religious High Council Under the Directorate of Religious Affairs (RHCDRA). *Günümüz tıp dünyasında tartışılan tüp bebek ve kök hücre gibi yeni uygulamaların İslam dini açısından değerlendirilmesi* [An assessment of the modern research on IVF and stem cells from an Islamic perspective]. Available at: www2.diyanet.gov.tr/dinisleriyuksekkurulu/Sayfalar/Tupbebek1023-5894.aspx (in Turkish). [Accessed 15 April 2015].

*Regulations on Patients' Rights*. In: *Official Gazette*, 1 August 1998, no. 23420. Available at: www.resmigazete.gov.tr/arsiv/23420.pdf (in Turkish). [Accessed 2 May 2015].

Rizvi, S. A. H., Naqvi, S. A. A., *et al.* 2004. Embryonic Stem Cell Research: An Islamic Standpoint. In: Gutmann, T., Daar, A. S., Sells, R. A., Land, W. (eds.). *Ethical, Legal and Social Issues in Organ Transplantation*. Lengerich: Pabst Science Publ., 391–9.

Royan Institute. *Reproductive Biomedicine and Stem Cell*. Available at: www.royaninstitute.org/. [Accessed 10 April 2015].

Sachedina, A. 2009. *Islamic Biomedical Ethics: Principles and Application*. Oxford: Oxford University Press.

Sahih Al Bukhari. 2002. *Dar Al-Risalah*. Beirut, Lebanon.

Saniei, M. and De Vries, R. 2008. Embryonic Stem Cell Research in Iran: Status and Ethics. *Indian Journal of Medical Ethics* 5(4), 181–4.

Saniei, M. 2012. Human Embryonic Stem Cell Research in Iran: The Significance of the Islamic Context. In: Inhorn, M. C. and Tremayne, S. (eds.). *Islam and Assisted Reproductive Technologies: Sunni and Shia Perspectives.* New York: Berghahn Books, 194–220.

Schienberg, J. and Katz, N. 2009. Iran: The Stem Cell Fatwa. *Frontline.* Available at: www.pbs.org/frontlineworld/rough/2009/06/iran_stem_cell.html. [Accessed 22 December 2009].

Serour, G. I. and Omran, A. R. (eds.). 1992. *Ethical Guidelines for Human Reproduction Research in the Muslim World: Based on Highlights, Papers, Discussions, and Recommendations of the First International Conference on Bioethics in Human Reproduction Research in the Muslim World, Cairo, 10–13 December, 1991.* Cairo: International Islamic Center for Population Studies and Research, Al-Azhar University, 30–1.

Serour, G. I. 1997. Islamic Developments in Bioethics, In: Lustig, B. A. (ed.). *Bioethics Yearbook, Volume 5: Theological Developments in Bioethics, 1992–1994.* Dordrecht: Springer, 171–88.

Sert, G., Güven, T. and Görkey, Ş. 2011. *Medical Law in Turkey.* Alphen (NL): Kluwer Law International, 30.

Shaltūt, M. 1971. *Al-Islām, 'aqīda wa Sharī'a.* [*Islam: Belief and Shari'a*]. Beirut: Dār ash-shurūq.

Siddiqi, M. 2002. An Islamic Perspective on Stem Cell Research. Available at: www.islamicity.com/articles/Articles.asp?ref=IC0202-404. [Accessed 10 June 2008].

Stavropoulos-Giokas, C., Charron, D. and Navarrete, C. (eds.). 2014. *Cord Blood Stem Cell Medicine.* San Diego: Elsevier (Academic Press), 259, 278.

Turkish Ministry of Health. 2014. Legislation Concerning the Practices of Assisted Reproduction Treatment Centers. In: *Official Gazette*, 30 September 2014, no. 29135. Available at: www.resmigazete.gov.tr/eskiler/2014/09/20140930.htm (in Turkish). [Accessed 2 May 2016].

Turkish Drug and Medical Device Institution. *Regulations on Clinical Trials of Drugs and Biological Products.* In: Official Gazette, 25 June 2014, no. 29041. Available at: www.resmigazete.gov.tr/eskiler/2014/06/20140625.htm (in Turkish). [Accessed 2 May 2015].

Tebourski, F. and Ammar-Elgaaied, A. B. 2004. The Developing Country Reaction to Biomedical Techniques and Plant Biotechnology: The Tunisian Experience. *Journal of Biomedicine and Biotechnology* 3, 124–9.

Turkish Ministry of Health. General Directorate of Healthcare Services. 2005. *Circular Note of Turkish Ministry of Health on Embryonic Stem Cell Research*, circular no. 2005/141. Available at: www.ttb.org.tr/mevzuat/index. php?option=com_content&task=view&id=347&Itemid=35 (in Turkish). [Accessed 2 May 2015].

Turkish Ministry of Health. General Directorate of Healthcare Services. 2006. *Circular Note of Turkish Ministry of Health on Stem Cell Studies*, Circular no. 2006/51. Available at: www.ttb.org.tr/mevzuat/index.php?option=com_conte nt&task=view&id=387&Itemid=35 (in Turkish). [Accessed 2 May 2015].

Walters, L. 2004. Human Embryonic Stem Cell Research: An Intercultural Perspective. *Kennedy Institute of Ethics Journal*, 14(1), 3–38.

*Washington Times*. 2009. Iran at Forefront of Stem Cell Research. Available at: www.washingtontimes.com/news/2009/apr/15/iran-at-forefront-of-stem-cell-research/. [Accessed March 15, 2016].

Weisser, U. 1983. *Zeugung, Vererbung und pränatale Entwicklung in der Medizin des arabisch-islamischen Mittelalters*. [*Procreation, Heredity, and Prenatal Development in the Medicine of the Arab-Islamic Middle Ages*]. Erlangen: Lüling.

Yeprem, S. 2006a. İslâm'ın kök hücreye bakışı. *Diyanet Aylık Dergi* 191, 25–9.

Yeprem, S. 2006b. Tüp bebek ve kök hücre gibi uygulamaların İslam dini açısından değerlendirilmesi. *Diyanet Aylık Dergi* 186, 29–32.

Yeprem, S. 2007. Die Haltungen der Religionen zu Gentechnologie, Sterbehilfe und Organtransplantationen. In: *Der Islam und das Christentum — Ein Vergleich der Grundwerte für einen interreligiösen Dialog*. Ankara: Konrad-Adenauer-Stiftung, 195–201.

# CHAPTER EIGHT

## Environmental Ethics in Islam

### *Azizan Baharuddin and Mohd Noor Musa*

### Summary

Muslims constitute one quarter of the earth's population and there are possibilities that Muslims can contribute to alleviate the environmental crisis currently faced. One important element of the transformational process is reaffirming the understanding among Muslims themselves of the value of nature or the environment. In Islam, nature caters to the spiritual and material needs of mankind. In the Qur'anic perspective, humans are created to serve the Creator which actually means to serve the highest good for oneself, the community, and the environment. This perspective is part of the foundation of Islamic environmental ethics. The attitude of gratitude or having the predisposition of being grateful (*shakur*) is also the basis for an environmentally moral stand. Based on these Islamic teachings, a Muslim is able to focus on his goal of resisting extremes in worldly temptations which often translate into environmentally wasteful and exploitative habits. In Islam, nature has its own order and functions (*fitrah*) that work naturally within ecosystems wherein the components are mutually dependent on each other. Any single disturbance will affect the balance (*mizan*) of the greater system and cause harm (*fasad*) to at least one or more components. To sustain the balance is a core principle of Islamic worldviews, which is to preserve and sustain the wellbeing of nature and to bring peace to its inhabitants. Such sustaining principles are enshrined in the philosophy of the objective of the Islamic law (*maqasid al-shariah*) and are explained in the Qur'an and *hadith*, the primary sources of guidance for Muslims. The scientific and/or empirical knowledge of the "what and how" of nature, as well as clarification of the responsibilities that humans have regarding the nature, are critical for the enforcement of Islamic environmental ethics.

## Introduction: Status of Environment in Islam

For Muslims, nature and its resources are bounties gifted from God to Man. The Qur'an describes and glorifies nature and wildlife as an earthly heaven; a mirror of the forests, gardens, and rivers of Paradise above. It is a major sign of the Mercy of the Creator, as He declares in the Qur'an "Do you not see that God has subjected to your use all things in the heavens and on the earth and has made his bounties flow to you in exceeding measures, seen and unseen?" (31: 20). Environmental ethics is critical in Islam because, as part and parcel of his well-being, Man needs to appreciate the bounties of God and strive to not wrong (*kufr*) them. Muslims constitute one quarter of the earth's population and with this attitude of gratitude Muslims could make many significant contributions in the world to alleviate the environmental crisis currently faced. An important element of the transformational process is the understanding of what nature or the environment are, and the imperative of *shakur* or gratefulness. The underlying meaning and purpose of gratefulness is expressed as follows:

> It is Allah Who created the heavens and the earth and sent down rain from the skies, and with it brought out fruits wherewith to feed you; it is He Who has made the ships subject to you, that they may sail through the sea by His command; and the rivers (also) He has made subject to you. And He has made subject to you the sun and the moon, both diligently pursuing their courses; and the night and the day have He (also) made subject to you. And He gives you of all that you ask for. But if you count the favours of Allah, never will you be able to number them. Verily, man is given up to injustice and ingratitude (14:32–34).

## Islamic Worldview on the Environment

According to Islam, nature has its own natural order that is regarded as the manifestation of acts of Allah (*sunnatullah*). Every element has been set to have its own functions. However, each element also is in relation with and needs other elements and is likewise "needed" by other elements; hence the notion of an ecosystem wherein the components are mutually dependent on each other. Any disturbance incurred on this order will cause harm to at least one component and to a certain extent to all other elements as well. This characteristic of nature is part of the fundamental knowledge of the vicegerent (*khalifah*), managing the environment with prudence and wisdom. More holistically, to be an effective vicegerent, one needs a clear worldview of the environment. Some principles of this worldview include the following:

— The universe is a sign of greatness and a proof of oneness of Allah. As decreed in the Qur'an: "Behold! In the creation of the heavens and the earth and the alternation of the night and the day, there are indeed signs for men of understanding" (3:190).
— The environment as a whole is a creation, and is novel (i.e., creation is constantly being renewed). Therefore nature is dependent on an external power and is exposed to changes as in growth and decay or decomposition. In fact, destruction is something that is inevitable and only Allah lasts.
— The environment exists as an order: any abuse, contamination, and imbalance in one component will impact other components.
— No creation has been created to be useless because the Creator is Most Wise, and did not create something that is purposeless. Every creation has its own function and use, whether it is already/will be known or not by humans.
— The environment is entrusted as a trust (*amanah*) to mankind as a whole. Therefore, it is an instrument to do good deeds, and this *amanah* should be a goal in itself.
— The environment is also a gift from the Creator that needs to be appreciated and we should be grateful for it. Thus, it needs to be taken care of and used as well as possible. Any form of waste and misuse is a form of ungratefulnessof the blessings given by Allah.

In Islamic environmental ethics, mankind carries the mission of *imarah* (to prosper) the gift of nature, synonymized as mentioned, as trust. It can be surmised therefore that one of the central missions of mankind on earth is to preserve and sustain the wellbeing of nature to bring peace to its inhabitants (both humans and non-humans). Therefore, it is perhaps appropriate to acknowledge that Islam's ultimate focus is to highlight the harmony in the interaction between man and the environment which essentially is the meaning of environmental ethics. One important way that man relates to Allah (in actual fact does so even though he is unaware of it) is via obedience to His way (*Shari'a*). This obedience is manifested in the mode he relates to other individuals in the context of serving social needs and social justice. Extended to the context of nature, man is neither a conqueror nor captor who desires to exploit everything around him as much as possible. Man is not and cannot be a slave in this temporary and worldly life. Even though he is given command and advantage over nature by virtue of the reason (*'aqal*), such "power" in reality is a test upon him. Nevertheless his possible failure in the trust given to him in fact is anticipated in the Qur'an in the following verse:

Mischief (corruption) has appeared on land and sea because of (the deed) that the hands of men have earned, that (Allah) may give them a taste of some of their deeds: in order that they may turn back (from evil) (30:51).

Reflection on this verse (*ayat*) is critical today as the *Islamic Declaration on Climate Change* at the end of the chapter indicates, in order to observe in greater detail the basic structure of the foundation of Islamic teaching regarding the environment, it is necessary to reflect seriously upon the Qur'an in the context of today's knowledge. The term the Qur'an uses to describe our natural surroundings is *khalq* (creation). It is estimated that the word *khalq* is mentioned significantly 261 times in the Qur'an (Mangunjaya 2013). Even the very first revelation of the Qur'an contains the verb *khalaq* (created): "Read! In the name of your Lord and Cherisher, Who created" (96:1). In a broader sense, man is part of the totality of the creational process and the Qur'an is the manual that lays down the foundation for the guideline (*Shari'a*) of our conduct in the affairs between man and man, and man and nature.

The term *Shari'a* — is also often understood as the detailed code of conduct, basis, or guidelines for ethics, morality, and laws that prescribe judgment of right and wrong (Mawdudi 2010). *Shari'a*, which derives from the Arabic word S*hara'a*, means the clear path, way, or the road to a watering place (nourishing for life). It clearly indicates the relationship between *Shari'a* and the environmental elements, notably water (*al-ma'*) and river water for example, was mentioned 63 and 52 times respectively ('Abdul Baqi 1987). Since there is no life without water, similarly there is no life without *Shari'a* (Nurdeng 2012). The objectives of the *Shari'a* (*maqasid al-Shari'a*) consist of five essential values namely: preservation and protection of faith; life; intellect; property; and lineage. Protection and maintenance of the environment via an Islamic environmental ethic will certainly protect faith, property, life, intellect and lineage.

The two principal sources of *Shari'a*, the Qur'an and the *Sunna*, are considered as a reflection of divine ethics. In the eyes of *Shari'a*, human action is not only categorized into good or bad, rather it is divided into five categories namely obligatory (*wajib*), recommended (*mandub*), neutral (*mubah*), discouraged (*makruh*), and prohibited (*haram*) because it causes harm (Zaidan 2001). The ultimate goal of *Shari'a* is blessing for mankind and the promotion of victory (*falaah*) or real well-being of all the people living on earth (Chapra 2008). The Islamic approach with regard to the environment is neither ecocentrism nor anthropocentrism *per se*. It strives to create a just balance between the rights and obligations of humans and those of His fellow creatures. Environmental ethics in Islam is better understood in a theocentric sense as God is the Creator (*al-Khaliq*) and Sustainer (*Al-Razzaq*). Indeed, Man is given dominance over nature. Yet, nature is not his to do as he pleases without limits. Nature contains "signs" of and from Allah. These signs are to be read and studied by human being so that he may overcome the temporary veil imposed upon him when he is placed on his earthly abode. The Qur'an describes the original declaration of faith of Muslim in the following verse:

When your Lord drew forth from the Children of Adam — from their loins — their descendants, and made them testify concerning themselves, (saying): "Am I not your Lord (who cherishes and sustains you)?" They said: "Yea! We do testify!" (This), lest ye should say on the Day of Judgment: "Of this we were never mindful" (7:172).

Emphasizing the critical importance of nature and man's knowledge and understanding of it, the verses in the Qur'an are descriptions of the orderliness, functions of the environment, and nature which scientists believe are in a state of contingency, that is, nothing can explain why the "forces" that keep nature (and the universe, for that matter) stable unless there is a super intelligence doing it. For Muslims, such a hypothesis is based on empirical evidence which points to the truth of God's existence. However, the Qur'an in the following verse does not ask Muslims to make enemies of those who do not accept the God hypothesis: "To you be your Way, and to me mine" (109:6).

In short, Islam has underlined human relations with the environment. Plants and animals for example are substantial beings that always interact with and have a big contribution to human life. In the Qur'an, flora is given a special attention and specific chapters are even named after plant or animal life, such as *At-Tin* (the fig tree) and *Al-Naml* (ant). Furthermore, there are numerous Qur'anic verses that mention human interaction with the environment; e.g 16:12; 6:141; 21:78. Islam also stresses several principles related to human interaction with flora and fauna exhorting "lessons" that humans should draw from their existence and functions. As will be further explained, Islamic environmental ethics is a balance between ecocentricism and anthropocentrism. Its "theocentric base" (empirically verifiable) allows it to keep a balance between these two. Islamic environmental ethics would not be alien to the life-centred worldview, described in the next section.

## Worldviews on the Environment

As mentioned, Islamic environmental ethics strives to strike a balance between a Man-centred worldview and extreme ecocentrism. Let us examine these two worldviews.

### *Man-centered worldview*

The separation between science and religion has caused the peripheralisation of values, meanings, and purposes. However, the importance of the demarcation of "rights" and "wrongs" that affect all areas of life provides the basis for the currently dominating Man-centered worldview (MCW).

The MCW, also known as the "planetary management worldview," has been the most dominant in the last 70 years (Baharuddin 2013). Miller (2004), for example, explains this worldview as being the most dominant in industrial societies of today. According to this MCW:

— We are the planet's most important species; we live apart from and are in charge of nature.
— There are always more (resources) and they are all for us.
— All forms of economic growth are good.
— A healthy environment depends on a healthy economy.
— Our success depends on how well we can understand, control, and manage the planet for our benefit.
— Other species have instrumental value only.
— As the most dominant species, man can and should manage planet for his benefit alone.

From the standpoint of ecological knowledge, it can be argued that the proponents of MCW are ignorant of the inappropriateness of such a chauvinistic stance towards nature. The Islamic perspective would inevitably not be in line with this approach.

### Life-centered worldview: working with the planet

It has been argued that the Life-Centered Worldview (LCW) is closer to reality and it is in harmony with many spiritually-based, empirically-verifiable belief systems of western as well as non-western societies in the world (Baharuddin 2013). This outlook has been illustrated by Miller (2004) in his efforts in the last three decades to put forward the new "sustainable" worldview. The increasing success of this new worldview is shown perhaps by the fact that his book *Living in the Environment* has been through 17 editions, the latest in 2012. From the Islamic perspective or the perspective of those whose indigenous philosophies speak for living in harmony with the environment, the LCW principles are already inherent in their sacred texts and teachings (Baharuddin 2013). Some of the principles of LCW are:

— Nature exists for all of earth's species.
— There will not always be more, and not all resources are for us.

— Some forms of economic growth are beneficial, some harmful.
— A healthy economy depends on a healthy environment.
— Our success depends on learning to cooperate with one another and with the rest of nature.
— Other species have a right to exist regardless of whether they have/do not have commercial/instrumental value.
— Man may be the most important species in terms of having reason, but he is also a moral–ethical being and his ethical decision-making framework should be extended to other species as well.

In the Islamic view however, the actual practices of Muslims may not match the environmental ideals spoken by the sacred texts. This may be because of the lack of "context" when religious principles are taught. The LCW is an example of such a context. This is one of the important arguments for the value of empiricising the meaning of religion. Likewise, imbuing the environment with a sense of respect, awe, humility, and responsibility (duty-based ethics) towards nature would go a long way in spiritualizing science as has been the practice since the Golden Age of the Islamic civilization. Therefore, here we see the need for the religiously motivated individuals to be acquainted with the LCW and the scientific evidence that lies behind the worldview of environmental ethics, which teachings already exist in the Islamic tradition.

## Islamic Principles of Environmental Ethics

From the perspective of the Islamic worldview, environmental ethics in Islam caters to spiritual and material needs. Its main goal is to seek the pleasure of Allah and such an attitude will affect the psycho-emotional and mental makeup of individuals by making them mentally strong. Equipped with this strength, mankind is able to focus on his goal of resisting extreme worldly temptations. It is essential to discuss the conceptual basis or foundational ideas governing a Muslims' worldview of the environment. Three aspects of Islamic life which govern a Muslim's worldview are: environmental consciousness, simplicity, and empathy for fellow created beings which have an important bearing on the maintenance of environmental balance (Akhtar 1996).

Principles of Islamic environmental ethics can be drawn from several sources. Apart from the Qur'an and *hadith*, environmentally sustaining practices as well as the many "green technologies" invented and used by the Muslim scientists, architects, builders, and farmers throughout the geographical areas (such as in Andalusia) have been recorded within the Golden Age of Islam. Beyond their descriptive studies of animals, plants, rocks, and mountains, Muslim natural historians were also studying both the symbolic significance of the natural world and the lessons man can learn morally and spiritually from the study of the natural order (Nasr 1976). The unity, vicegerency, servanthood, balance, nature, trust, and human accountability are major values which shape Islamic perspectives in environmental ethics.

## Unity (*tawhid*)

The basis of Islam is *tawhid* (monotheism, singularity, oneness or unity of God) which is the most cardinal principle of Islamic faith and affects every Islamic approach especially environmental ethics. It implies that the whole universe is created, controlled and sustained by One Supreme Being. It informs relationships between God and man, man and man, and man and nature. The relationships highlight that all parts of the universe are created by the One God, Allah. *Tawhid* is the most fundamental of Islamic teachings and is the first principle of the five pillars of Islam. The affirmation of this fact marks the Muslim's declaration of faith (Shah Haneef 2002). *Tawhid* signifies one's belief in the oneness of God Who alone is the creator, sustainer, and provider of all life, as Qur'an reads:

> Allah — there is no god but He, the Living, the Self-Subsisting, Supporter of all. No slumber can seize Him nor sleep. His are all things in the heavens and on earth. Who is thee can intercede with His presence except as His permmitteth? He knows what is [presently] before them and what will be after them, and they encompass not a thing of His knowledge except for what He wills. His (throne) extends over the heavens and the earth, and their preservation tires Him not. And He is the Most High, the Most Great (2:255).

The concept of *tawhid* if properly understood plays a paramount role in creating order and consistency in a Muslim's thinking and behavior especially where he affects the environment as described below:

— Within the *tawhidic* world view, man is duty bound to live in harmony with the ecosystem, and in "maintaining" this harmony he is glorifying God.
— "The seven heavens and the earth and whatever is in them exalt Him. And there is not a thing except that it exalts [Allah] by His praise, but you do not understand their [way of] exalting. Indeed, He is ever Forbearing and Forgiving" (17: 44).
— Every creature and element of the ecosystem has an assigned role, whose loss and extinction if not remedied is bound to result in environmental crisis.
— The belief of a Muslim about the knowledge of God both of secret and open of things perpetually makes him do what is good and avoid what is wrong. This kind of awareness saves him from irresponsible and cruel use of nature and its destruction (Shah Haneef 2002).

### Vicegerency (khalifah)

The Qur'anic term *khalifah* originates from the word *khalafah* — which means to succeed or to replace a person either due to his absence or his incompetence, or as an honor to the successor. In the Islamic view, human beings were created as God's vicegerents on earth:

Behold," thy Lord said to the angels: "I will create a vicegerent on earth." They said: "Wilt Thou place therein one who will make mischief and shed blood? — whilst we do celebrate Thy praises and glorify Thy holy (name)?" He said: "I know what ye know not" (2:30).

The concept of vicegerency signifies the position of humans as the dwellers and occupiers of the earth who build a civilization on earth and inhabit whilst glorifying it. Madjid (1999) stated that in serving his responsibility as a guardian, man must know some facts and realities:

— Man's dignity in the context of his vicegerency reflects the consciousness that he indeed, at least in the physical sense, is likewise indebted

to nature for providing him not only with what he needs; but nature is indeed as well the means for him to do his good deeds.
— This dignity is also related to the universal values of humanity.
— To carry out his duties as God's guardian of the earth, man needs to have scientific knowledge.
— Although man's dignity is highlighted by his freedom, the latter comes with restrictions.
— Any breach of the limits degrades natures and man himself.
— The impulse to breach the limit is called greed, i.e., the unquenchable feeling that all the gifts from God are inadequate; it can be neutralized by the practice of *shukur*.
— Direction from God is required as a spiritual safety net as science alone does not explain the absence of a guarantee that man will not fall into degradation.

In managing the earth, man the *khalifah* is expected to act based on knowledge/science and not his own desire, (4:135; 23:71), as the lack of such knowledge will allow greed to breed resulting not only in short-term but also in long-term losses (Mangunjaya 2013). Men are expected to keep their pledge as *khalifah* while carrying out their mandate, as Allah has said:

> We did indeed offer the trust to the heavens and the earth and the mountains; but they refused to undertake it, being afraid thereof; but man undertook it: he was indeed unjust and foolish (33:72).

### Servanthood (*ubudiyyah*)

The word *ubudiyyah* is derived from the root word of *'abd* (slave), which literally means the state of slavery or servanthood (Ibnu Manzur 1995). In Islamic teaching, it refers to the highest and most praiseworthy human condition when he voluntarily believes in God and surrenders himself to Him alone, by doing his bidding outwardly and inwardly (Shah Haneef 2002). The religious impulse of doing things for the sake of God alone tremendously motivates Muslims to initiate and undertake constructive and good works for the benefit of humans which include serious concern and care for nature, the ecosystem, and the proper handling of its resources for human well-being. Also, responsibility to save the environment is part of the servanthood — act of submission — to God (*'ibadah*) in Islam.

## Balance (*mizan*)

The idea of balance has been highly prioritized and assessed in conservation efforts (Rockström *et al. 2009*). Al Gore (1992) recorded that man releases 90 million tons of carbon dioxide every day. To balance this, it would take forests and oceans from 30 to 1,000 years to absorb these emissions. Global warming is therefore directly caused by man's destruction of balance through the pollution of the air with greenhouse gases. This destruction of balance is thus considered to be anthropogenic, or created by man.

*Mizan*, according to the word's origin, means "scale" or "balance." Allah provides a fundamental picture in the Qur'an that depicts the creation of a balanced heaven and earth, in which everything in the universe is created in pairs (36:36). Allah said "And the firmament has He raised high, and He has set up the balance in order that you may not transgress (due) balance" (55:7–8). Yet, Allah the Almighty has established a very precise standard for human beings: "Verily, all things have [We] created in proportion and measure" (16:49).

Precise and accurate measures ensure the equilibrium of life on Earth, and as God created the world according to balance, the teachings of Islam are also based on balance and justice. Even the mind and conscience of man are created in harmony with its teachings. Therefore one should not lean too far to the right or to the left, but instead strive to achieve balance in all aspects of life (Mangunjaya 2013).

## Nature (*fitrah*)

*Fitrah* literally means "origin", "originality", or a "natural state." In its proper definition, *fitrah* is a "natural state or instinct that is found in man, animals, or something that compels man or any creature to require such state." Muslims are born in a state of purity. Islamic scholars agree with Naess (2005) and his eight basic principles of deep ecology which state that everything in life should happen naturally. The creations and functions for each species are important to allow evolution of the species. Al-Faruqi (1980) relies on the causality and effects of the juncture where the uniformity of nature has been affected by the law of nature. For example, natural events happen as consequences of a variety of causes, and they in turn act as causes producing further consequences. Orderliness and uniformity contribute to the influence of incongruity in the creation of the Beneficent Allah (67:3–4). Completeness will continue to be a feature of the natural world as long as it exists because Allah's creation always remains the same and the rules of nature are enduring (Setia 2003).

In accordance with the idea that it has been created perfect, each creature in nature is given an essence, a structure which determines its life and from which it never deviates (Al-Faruqi 1980). On the other hand, God never acts arbitrarily and his *Sunna* (laws and pattern) are immutable (30:30). In cases in which those created beings have been granted a certain degree of freedom, they exercise this freedom within a specific field by aligning themselves with or against their *fitrah,* i.e. the original divine pattern on which they have been created (if they have the freedom to do so, such as in the case of mankind) (Iqbal 2006).

### Trust and human accountability (amanah)

Trust (*amanah*) is the main responsibility of man particularly after he has agreed to shoulder the task of vicegerency offered to him by God, as explained earlier.

> We did indeed offer the trust to the heavens and the earth and the mountains. But they refused to undertake it, being afraid thereof; but man undertook it — he was indeed unjust and foolish (ignorant that some may betray it) (33:72).

According to the above Qur'anic verse, the trust given to man as a vicegerent is to build up a civilization for the good of all humanity and its environment as is willed by God. *Amanah* also means being honest and sincere in doing things and keeping safe from doing things prohibited (*haram*) by God. Technically, *amanah* is ensuring one's rights and responsibilities in relation to God or fellow humans or even other creatures, in work, words, and belief (Laming 1995). In terms of its application, it practically stands for fulfilling one's responsibility in all dimensions of life and relationships, as declared by The Prophet of Islam in a *hadith*:

> Every one of you is a guardian (leader) and everyone will be asked about his subjects; the leader is a guardian. He will be asked about his subjects. A man is the guardian of the persons in his household. He is answerable about his duties to them. A woman is the guardian of her husband's house. She will be asked about her responsibility. The servant is the guardian of the articles of his master. He is answerable about his responsibility over these (Bukhari Vol. 9, Book 89, Judgment No: 252).

The *hadith* precisely outlines the all-embracing dimensions and application of the trust inherent in life. There are other ample examples from the Qur'an and the *Sunna* which specifically address other applied instances of *amanah* in a Muslim's life, both personal and social. As for its application to the environment — humans (individually and collectively) are responsible for safekeeping the environment. The reason is that man has been made the master (without its negative connotations) over nature and its resources; and is held accountable and responsible for maintaining and preserving it, as stated in the Qur'an:

> And who created the species, all of them, and has made for you of ships and animals those which you mount. That you may settle yourselves upon their backs and then remember the favor of your Lord when you have settled upon them and say, "Exalted is He who has subjected this to us, and we could not have [otherwise] subdued it. And indeed we, to our Lord, will [surely] return" (43:12–14).

If a human fails to fulfill this *amanah*, he will be committing *khiyanah* which designates betrayal of trust — a kind of hypocrisy. The crime of *khiyanah* and *fasaad* [*corruption*] committed against the environment is so enormous that it brings man and nature to the brink of annihilation, thus amounting to self-destruction which is categorically prohibited (*haram*) in Islam, as Qur'an reads: "And make not your hands contribute to your destruction; but do good; for God loveth those who do good" (2:195).

## Islamic Measures and Recommendations to Protect the Environment

There are several recommendations (as principles) in the Qur'an and *hadith* which encourage human beings to protect the environment.

### Protection of animals and plants

Plants and animals are important components of the environment. As part of God's creation like other living organisms, they have their assigned role to play, especially in terms of facilitating the proper environmental conditions for humans. Air is filtered by plant life for animal use, in return animals exhale carbon dioxide to be utilized by plants for photosynthesis. The Qur'an reminds Muslims that everything in the universe has a role and no creature is without an assigned place in the cosmos. Allah says in the Qur'an:

> Those who remember Allah while standing or sitting or [lying] on their sides and give thought to the creation of the heavens and the earth, [saying], "Our Lord, You did not create this aimlessly; exalted are You [above such a thing]; then protect us from the punishment of the Fire" (3 191).

Islam also prohibits cutting, shearing or causing plants to die without a reasonable cause or excuse; deforestation is not encouraged. The Prophet also tells us to restore the wetland and revive the dead land, as he encouraged Muslims by saying:

> No Muslim, who plants a shoot, except that whatever is eaten or stolen from it, or anyone obtains the least thing from it, is considered like paying charity on his behalf until the day of judgment (Al Tirmidhi 1985).

It was in line with the above that Abu Bakr, the first caliph of Islam, strictly prohibited the unnecessary destruction of plants even during a military campaign. Also, the Prophet stresses the need to protect and conserve the green state of the environment, in its natural form; "This world is beautiful and green and Allah has made you His representatives on it and He sees (all things)" (Narrated by Muslims).

Islam is also very particular about human interactions with animals. The Qur'an itself includes the names of animals as the title of some chapters such as *Al-An'am* (farm animals), *Al-Nahl* (bees), *Al-Baqarah* (calf), *An-Naml* (ants), *Al-'Ankabut* (spider), and *Al-Fil* (elephant). Human interaction with fauna is further described in the Qur'an in several verses such as; 23:80, 6:142, 36:71–73. The narrated history (*seerah*) of the Prophet's time even describes the consequence of being sent to hell if a person abuses a cat, while another person is rewarded with heaven because of his good deeds to a dog. These confirm the significance of human interaction with animals.

### Saving land, water and air

The modern lifestyles of man have led to the insensitive use of resources, such as water, besides causing immense problems of environmental pollution. The Islamic measures to save land, air and water pollution are well governed by the principle of purification (*taharah*) — a central position in the teaching of Islam that makes the avoidance of pollutants (natural or chemical) an integral part of the Islamic faith: "And God loves those who make themselves clean and pure" (9:108). The Prophet also declares that purification is a branch of faith and God is supremely clean and loves those who uphold cleanliness (Al-Tirmidhi 1985, 107). To put the above imperatives in place in practice, the Prophet enacted the following:

— Do not pollute the water. As we read: "None of you must pass urine in still water which does not flow and then take a bath therein" (Al-Tirmidhi 1985, 200).
— Do not dispose of natural waste on the earth. As he said: "Beware of the two acts that bring curses: passing a stool in the path of people or in the shade of the trees" (Narrated by Abi Davoud).

Also, he pronounced an edict requiring the dead to be buried deep inside the earth so as to prevent not only fouling the atmosphere but also bacterial outbreaks when he said: "Dig a grave deep enough for a man's height and make it broader" (Karim 1994).

By analogy, the above examples of measures of the Prophet to protect the natural environment from being polluted by natural pollutants can be extended to cover all contemporary forms of toxic and chemical pollutants which are even more hazardous and offensive.

### Protection of other natural resources

Making a loud noise is unethical, rude and impolite. As the Qur'an says: "and lower thy voice; for the harshest of sounds without doubt is the braying of the ass" (31:19).

In order to teach his followers the "law" on noise pollution, whenever he sneezed, the Prophet used to cover his face with his hand or with a cloth so as to drown the sound of his voice therewith (Al-Tirmidhi 1985, 103). It is *haram* (prohibited) to inflict harm on others by disturbing their quiet and today we know that the sneeze can also allow contagious diseases to spread. This is an Islamic principle that was laid out in the *hadith*: "harm must neither be inflicted nor reciprocated" (Al Qazvini 2007, 39).

So even if the sound of sneezing might be deemed insignificant, so fine was the *akhlaq* (ethics) of the Prophet, that even a sneeze was considered a part of one's personal ethics.

## Islam and Environment: Going Green through Religion

As mentioned earlier, the following verse is currently highlighted more and more.

> Mischief has appeared on land and sea because of (the greed) that the hands of men have earned, that (Allah) may give them a taste of some of their deeds: in order that they may turn back (from evil) (30:41).

By now there is a consensus that the environmental crisis, such as climate change, is largely a man-made phenomenon. Some would even be more forthright in saying it is a self-inflicted wound and its effects may be irreversible. Life could become (or has become) very difficult for some plants, animals, and humans. Not only species and resources but cultures too could be lost and are being lost. The greatest challenge we currently face in addressing climate change is our lack of proper awareness and ineffective collective efforts in arresting climate change or even just slowing it down. For communities of faith, doing something to safeguard the environment is part of their religious duty. Any alternative theories of environmental ethics or worldviews regarding the environment can therefore be expected to challenge the basic proposition of the dominant modern understanding and worldview of nature to find the best solution for this crisis. In the United States for example, Sayed Hasan Nasr wrote *Man and Nature: The Spiritual Crisis in Modern Man* in 1968 and is regarded by some as the first green Muslim. Nasr stresses the importance of a greater awareness of the origins of both man and nature as a means of righting the imbalance that exists in our deepest selves and in the environment. He highlights the observation that since the emergence of the environmental crisis, modern humans have begun to perceive religion from a new standpoint: from an ecological outlook in which everything is connected to everything else and nature is seen as an organic unity (Nasr 1968).

In view of these considerations, Islam provides ethical guidelines and clear teaching (as mentioned) on how Muslims should manage and glorify the earth. Therefore, it is the responsibility of every Muslim to act (*'amal*) following the Prophet Muhammad who is the best example and blessing for the whole world. Such ethical examples (*Sunna*) are stated in the *Islamic Declaration on Climate Change* (IDCC). The IDCC is a collective agreement by Muslim leaders, scholars, scientists, NGOs, and policy-makers who call on the world's 1.6 billion Muslims to do their part to eliminate dangerous greenhouse gas emissions and commit to using and creating renewable energy sources.[2] The declaration calls on Muslim countries — especially those that are "well-off" and "oil-producing" — to lead the change in phasing out greenhouse gas emissions. The declaration also calls on wealthy Muslim countries to provide financial and technical support to less-affluent states so they all can work to eliminate pollution; reduce consumption of finite resources; work to stabilize the Earth's temperature; abandon "unethical profit from the environment;" and help create a global green economy.

The declaration furthermore calls for action based on the good practice and examples demonstrated by the Prophet such as declaring and protecting the rights of all living beings; prohibiting the killing of living beings for sport; conserving water even in ablution (*wudhu'*) for prayer; forbidding the felling of trees in the desert; and establishing "inviolable geographic zones" (i.e. around Makkah and Al-Madinah). Within these zones native plants may not be felled or cut and wild animals may not be hunted or disturbed. The Prophet led a frugal life, free of excess, waste, and ostentation and he avoided over-consumption. The Prophet and his companions established protected areas (*himas*) for the conservation and sustainable use of land, plants, and wildlife. Several *himas* that still exist today can be found in the Middle East and Arab regions. *Hima* is considered unique by environmentalists as it is based upon communal leadership and is maintained by the surrounding communities (Mangunjaya 2013). Some other practical ways Islamic institutions can bring the green religion (*deen*) concepts to life include the examples of a collaboration by 500 mosques in Terengganu, Malaysia to present sermons on turtle conservation in 2008; and of the Leeds mosque in the United Kingdom posting on its website links to Islam and the environment and encouraging recycling activities on its premises. Similarly "green" *pesantrens* (religious schools) in Indonesia and other encouraging examples of "going green" are beginning to be seen all over the Muslim world. Muslims are encouraged to be involved in such ventures and to carry out activities that show its society (*jamaah*) practical green steps to follow such as water and energy saving methods; creating recycling systems; waste management; and green architecture as they bear in mind the words of our Prophet: "The world is sweet and verdant, and verily Allah has made you stewards in it, and He sees how you acquit yourselves."[3]

## Conclusion

The primary sources of guidance for Muslims in all areas are the Qur'an and the *Sunna* of the Prophet. The Qur'an is the direct Word of God and it contains over 650 references to ecology as well as important principles which are able to be applied to the environment. The sayings and actions of the Prophet (*Sunna* and *Hadith*) are the secondary source of guidance for Muslims. The Qur'an also contains numerous important ecological guidelines. In fact, there is an abundance of *hadith* concerning plants, trees, land cultivation, irrigation, crops, livestock, grazing, water distribution, and treatment of animals. The *Shari'a* law or the body of Islamic law sets the legal framework for applying the Qur'anic principles and guidelines of the Prophet Muhammad. In addition, many teachings explain how to apply these principles to public and private aspects of life. Collectively, the sources of authority in Islam provide very clear ethical teaching, worldview, and direction to Muslims in their relationship with the environment.

## Notes

1   See Al-Hassani, S. T. S., Woodcock, E. and Saoud, R. (eds.). 2007. *1001 Muslim Inventions: Muslim Heritage in Our World*. Manchester: Foundation for Science, Technology and Civilization (FSTC).

2   *Islamic Declaration on Climate Change* (IDCC) draws on Islamic teachings and was presented at Conference of Parties (COP21) in Paris where international negotiators was set to hash out a global plan to combat climate change. It was drafted by academics and finalized at the International Islamic Climate Change Symposium held in Istanbul on 17–18 August 2015. The symposium's goal was to reach broad unity and ownership from the Islamic community around the Declaration. It invites people of all nations and their leaders to join forces to fight climate change, supported by the grand *muftis* — interpreters of Islamic law — of Lebanon and Uganda, as well as other prominent Islamic scholars. See: http://islamicclimatedeclaration.org/islamic-declaration-on-global-climate-change/.

3   *Hadith* related by a Muslim from Abu Sa'īd Al-Khudrī. Also mentioned in the *Islamic Declaration on Climate Change* (IDCC).

## References

Abdul Baqi, M. F. 1987. *Al-Mu'jam al-Mufahras Li alfaz al-Qur'an al-Karim*. [*Dictionary of Qur'an*]. Cairo: Dar al-Hadith.

Akhtar, M. R. 1996. Towards an Islamic Approach for Environmental Balance. *Islamic Economic Studies*, 3(2), 57–76.

Al-Faruqi, I. R. 1980. *Islam and Culture*. Kuala Lumpur: Angkatan Belia Islam Malaysia (ABIM).

Al-Qazwini, M. B. Y. Ibn Majah, 2007. *Sunan Ibn Majah (Narrated Hadith)*. Tahir, Hafiz Abu and Za'i, Zubair 'Ali (eds.). Riyadh: Maktaba Dar-us-Salam.

Al-Tirmidhi, Muhammad ibn 'isa. 1985. *Sunan al-Tirmidhi, Volume 2 (Narrated Hadith)*. Karachi: Sa'id Publishing.

Amery, H. A. 2001. Islamic Water Management. *Water International*, 26(4), 482–8.

Azizan, B. 2013. Changing Our Worldview for a Sustainable Future and the Role of Dialogue. *Journal of Oriental Studies*, 23, 40–51.

Chapra, M. U. 2008. *The Islamic Vision of Development in the Light of the Maqasid al-Shari'ah*. Herndon: The International Institute of Islamic Thought.

Gore, A. 1992. *Earth in the Balance: Ecology and the Human Spirit*. Houghton Mifflin Harcourt.

Hammoud, M. 1990. Environment, Ecology and Islam. *Insight* (Islamic Foundation, NSW) 5(3).

Islamic Sciences and Research Academy (ISRA). 2013. *Environmental Ethics in Islam*. Available at: http://www.ceosyd.catholic.edu.au/Parents/Religion/Documents/20130715-doc-EnvironmentalEthicsIslam.pdf.

*Islamic Declaration on Climate Change*. 2015. International Islamic Symposium on Climate Change, 17–18 August. Istanbul: Islamic Relief Worldwide. Available at: http://islamicclimatedeclaration.org/islamic-declaration-on-global-climate-change/.

Iqbal, M. 2006. In the Beginning: Islamic Perspectives on Cosmological Origins. *Islam and Science*, 4(2), 93–112.

Karim, F. 1994. *Mishkat al-Masabih*. [*A Niche for Lamps*], 3rd ed. New Delhi: Islamic Book Service.

Kilani, H., Serhal, A. and Llewlyn, O. 2007. *Al-Hima: A Way of Life*. Amman: IUCN West Asia Regional Office. Available at: http://cmsdata.iucn.org/downloads/al_hima.pdf.

Laming, S. 1995. *Knowledge, Khilafah and Amanah in Islam*. Selangor: Ans Mega.

Madjid, N. 1999. *Cita-cita Politik Islam Era Reformasi*. [*The Islamic Political Idea of the Reform Era*]. Jakarta: Yayasan Wakaf Paramadina.

Mangunjaya, F. M. 2013. Islam and Natural Resource Management. In: MacKay, J. E. (ed.). *Integrating Religion within Conservation: Islamic Beliefs and Sumatran Forest Management*. Canterbury: Durrell Institute of Conservation and Ecology, University of Kent.

Mawdudi, A. A. 2010. *Towards Understanding Islam*. Rev. ed. Kuala Lumpur: Dar Al Wahi Publication, 150.

Miller, G. T. 2004. *Living in the Environment: Principles, Connections, and Solutions.* Pacific Grove, CA: Brooks/Cole-Thompson Learning.

Muhammad Ibn Mukrim Ibn Manzur. 1995. *Lisan al-Arab.* [*Arabic Language*]. Beirut: Dar Sadir.

Naess, A. 2005. The Basics of Deep Ecology. *The Trumpeter*, 21(1), 61–71.

Nasr, S. H. 1968. *Man and Nature: The Spiritual Crisis in Modern Man.* [n.p.]: ABC International Group.

Nasr, S. H. 1976. *Islamic Science: An Illustrated Study.* London: World of Islam Festival Publishing Company Limited.

Nurdeng, D. 2012. New Essential Values of *Daruriyyah* (Necessities) of the Objectives of Islamic Law (*Maqasid Al-Shari`ah*). *Jurnal Hadhari*, 4(2), 107–116.

Rockström, J. *et al.* 2009. A Safe Operating Space for Humanity. *Nature* 461, 472–5.

Setia, A. 2003. Al- Attas' Philosophy of Science. *Islam and Science*, 1(2), 166–213.

Shah Haneef, S. S. 2002. Principles of Environmental Law in Islam. *Arab Law Quarterly,* 17(3), 241–54.

Sulayman ibn Ah'ath. Undated. *Sunan Abi Davud.* Karachi: Kitab Khana Markaz 'ilm wa Adab.

Zaidan, A. K. 2001. *Al-Wajiz fi Usul al-Fiqh.* [*The Fundamentals of Islamic Jurisprudence*]. Beirut: Muassasah al-Risalah.

# CHAPTER NINE

## Animal Rights in Islam: The Use of Animals for Medical Research

### Bagher Larijani, Nazafarin Ghasemzadeh and Mansoureh Madani

### Summary

In Islam, there are numerous ethical recommendations regarding the proper treatment of animals. These recommendations are not purely based on human sentiments, or on utilitarian purposes, or on any financial benefits from the use of animals. Rather these recommendations are founded on the sanctity of animal life and the inherent rights of animals. These recommendations should be regarded as God's order to protect animals' physical rights and specifically to prohibit physical and psychological harassment of animals. In Islamic societies it is important to take Islamic points of view into account while using animals in medical sciences and research. Accordingly, while working with laboratory animals it is important to keep the following goals in mind: using the least number of animals; providing all appropriate care for animals, even animals that are dying; minimizing animal suffering and psychological abuse; as well as giving priority to safety and animal welfare. To assist in achieving these goals, regulations as well as legislation are necessary to ensure respect for the rights of laboratory animals. This chapter presents an Islamic perspective on animal rights and discusses some of the possible regulatory frameworks for the use of animals for research and education in biomedicine.

## Introduction

In the past, due to each era's common attitudes, animals were used without any restrictions. Philosophers such as Augustine considered animals solely as a tool to be used by humans, Descartes regarded animals to be like machines and without consciousness. Moreover, Kant believed that human beings have no responsibility toward animals because animals lack self-awareness (la Velle 2002). However, in the past few decades, increasing recognition of animals' rights has led to the imposition of restrictions in this area. The Islamic tradition has a long history of observing animal rights. According to Islamic teachings, using animals is permitted with a justified reason and any violent behavior towards animals is prohibited. Islam prohibits both physical and psychological abuse because animals possess wisdom and sensations. Thus, Islam calls for the humane, kind, and dignified treatment of animals. Moreover, not only animal owners, but also others, and especially the Islamic government are responsible for taking care of animals. In Islam, killing animals is primarily forbidden unless it is done for more important reasons authorized by God.

This chapter describes animal rights in Islam and refers to religious teachings instructing how to treat animals. It also discusses conditions in which laboratory animals can be used in biomedical research. It should be noted that regarding animal rights there are very minor differences between *Shi'ite* and *Sunni* jurisprudences.

## The Status of Animals in Islamic Context

The Qur'an introduces animals as a source of edification for humans and according to some Qur'anic verses, animals are considered as a source of comfort. There are also verses in the Qur'an that consider animals to possess an amount of wisdom that refer to some degree of resurrection of animals after death.

In this regards Qur'an reads:

And there is no creature on [or within] the earth or bird that flies with its wings except [that they are] communities like you. We have not neglected in the Register a thing. Then unto their Lord they will be gathered.(6:38)

And indeed, for you in livestock is a lesson. We give you drink from that which is in their bellies, and for you in them are numerous benefits, and from them you eat. (23:21)

In Islam, human beings and animals possess rights because they are alive. All rights in Islam are granted by God and the rightful owners can use their specific rights just by God's will. According to a number of Muslim jurists including the author of *Jawaher al-Kalaam*, an authoritative book in Islamic jurisprudence, an animal's right is equal to God's right. He has stated that if an animal's owner requests to stop feeding the animal, nobody should obey because God orders everyone to feed and treat animals kindly. If it is necessary — in the case of an abandoned animal — even the government should take care of animal needs (Najafi 1984, 111). It should be noted that the reason that Islam emphasizes the rights of animals is not for fear of economic loss, but is for the respect of the all living creatures that have a soul. According to Sheikh Tusi, animals should receive enough care and support since they are revered (Tusi 1968). Therefore, if an animal is thirsty and we have only enough water for ablution (*wudu*), for praying, we should give the water to the animal even if we know that it will not save the animal (Najafi 1984, 115) or when we are afraid of getting drowned in a ship, to decrease the weight of the ship, we must throw other belongings out of the ship and avoid animals' deaths as much as possible. Under that condition, one must not throw a living creature while there are still other material goods on the ship (Ameli-Shahid Thani 1993, 383). Another point that must be mentioned about animal rights in Islam is that these laws, unlike other laws about animals, are not solely motivated based on respect for human feelings and emotions, but are based on respecting the animal's life (Jafari Tabrizi 1999).

## Animal Rights in Islam

Islam respects animals as God's creatures and accordingly has instructed Muslims on how to treat animals. Islamic teachings emphasize providing for animals housing, food, clothing, medicine, sanitation, and all other requirements whether or not the animal is edible or profitable for its owner. Islam also prohibits any harassment of living animals such as shortening fingernails of the milker before milking an animal and avoiding the destruction of insect nests. The general rule is that ownership necessitates care and provisions of all the common needs which may differ depending on the conditions, even when an animal is dying. (Ameli-Shahid Thani 1990; Najafi 1984). This rule should also be applied to silkworms and honeybees. For instance, sufficient berry leaves and honey must be provided for the insects so that they do not feel hunger. Moreover, if milking an animal is hazardous for its health, for example, it is sick or has not eaten enough food then milking is forbidden (*haram*) (Najafi 1984, 396). It is is necessary not only to meet the animal's needs, but also that of their offspring. As long as the baby needs milk, milking the mother is forbidden unless the baby eats enough or it gets old enough to eat grass and forage to sustain itself (Tusi 1968; Najafi 1984, 396).

In case the owner does not obey these recommendations to treat animals kindly, the government must oblige him to provide monetary support or give the animal to another person. Saving an animal's life is also highly recommended. For instance, if the life of an animal is highly dependent on something like a piece of suture thread and somebody else has it, the animal owner should pay its price and save the animal's life (Hilli 1993). Even in case that the suture thread belongs to another individual who does not want to sell it and there is no other alternative to save the animal's life, some Islamic jurists recommend going to a judge to get help in saving the animal's life (Esfahani-Fazel Hendi 1996).

Sanitation must also be provided by the owner or the government in case the owner fails to do so. Islam supplies recommendations about the cleanliness of the food and animals' housing. For instance, it is quoted that the Prophet has ordered people to keep sheep in a clean place and wipe their noses (Horr Ameli 1989, 508; Kulayni 1987, 544). In another *hadith*, it is advised to wipe the noses of the sheep and say prayers in their fold (Horr Ameli 1989, 513). Moreover, the Prophet of Islam recommends people to clean their animals' food and states that if anyone cleans barley grains and gives them to his horse to relieve its hunger, God will reward him for every single barley grain that he has cleaned (Majlisi 1983, 177).

It is noteworthy that meeting all of an animal's requirements is considered mandatory (sufficing obligation or *wajib kifai*) for all, and all Muslims are responsible until someone has taken responsibility for the care of the animal (Ameli-Shahid Thani 1993, 251; Najafi 1984, 439). First and foremost, it is the responsibility of the Islamic government to monitor animal maintenance conditions. It is even mentioned that people who have put too much burden on an animal's back should be asked to put that burden on the ground if it bothers the animal (Montazeri Najaf Abadi 1989). In addition to the government, every individual has the duty to help an animal in need even if its owner forbids them to do so.

Other recommendations prohibit all kinds of disturbance and harassment of animals. This prohibition applies to all conscious creatures, even insects and aquatic animals, and addresses every annoyance, even very minor physical or psychological abuse.

Imam Sadiq (Sixth Shi'ite Imam), has forbidden praying next to ants' nests because it bothers or kills them (Hilli 1994). Moreover, Imam Sajjad advised his companions to avoid killing an animal at night since night provides a time for all creatures to relax (Horr Ameli 1989, 41). If a Muslim harasses his animal to arrive at Mecca for Hadj quickly, earlier than the others, Muslim leaders should not accept his testimony in court (Kulayni 1987, 396). In addition, there are numerous narratives that prohibit animal owners from putting too heavy burdens on animals (Kulayni 1987, 541). It is even advised that the burden be placed symmetrically on the animal so that it does not lean towards nor be seated to one side since it may injure the animal's back (Esfahani Majlesi-e Aval 1994). It is also stated that people should put the burden on the backside of the camel since its hind legs are stronger. It is also prohibited to seat several people on an animal's back. In another *hadith*, it is suggested that the rider feed his animal first and then himself when he has stopped to rest (Horr Ameli 1989, 479) and not to make the burden heavy on the animal. As well, it is stated that if three people sit on an animal, one of them is cursed (Horr Ameli 1989, 496). The person milking should maintain short fingernails so the animal is not annoyed (Najafi 1984, 307). Whipping animals, especially on the face, has been repeatedly prohibited. Quoting Imam Sajjad, it is stated that he had gone on 40 Hadj pilgrimages and had not whipped his camel even once (Qomi Sadugh 1993, 292–3). Even the use of offensive language is considered forbidden in Islam because it shows disrespect to a creature possessing consciousness. In a narrative from Imam Ali (First Shi'ite Imam), it is mentioned that if anyone curses an animal, he will be cursed by God (Qomi Sadugh 1993, 287).

Before Islam was embraced, violence was common towards animals. Islam repeatedly prohibits such violence as making animals fight with each other, sterilizing, mutilating, and killing animals in war, etc. Islamic narratives similar issues are forbidden (Moghimi Haji 2006).

Imam Ali orders tax collection officers to respect animal rights during shipment, and to choose a shepherd who is benevolent, honest, and caring. A shepherd who is not strict or unjust will not make them move too quickly and get overtired as a result. Whenever you give an animal to someone, ask him "to be just when riding camels. Care about an injured or tired camel. Take them near a source of water on the way. Let them rest sometime and eat grass and drink water when they arrive at the pasture...,these actions will reward you greatly and direct you, God willing" (Nahj al-Balaghah, Letter No. 25).

As was previously mentioned, killing animals is very blameworthy and is not permissible except for cases such as when a human is endangered or the animal will be used as food. In terms of consumption of meat, Islam recommends repeatedly that meat should be consumed sufficiently to ensure good health. Several *hadith* have recommended that eating meat more than three times in a day and less than once in 40 days is disliked (*makruh*) (Esfahani Majlesi-e Aval 1980). Thus, hunting for pleasure is forbidden (*haram*). However, hunting for the purpose of feeding humans is permissible only in particular conditions such as when the animal is slaughtered with a keen tool and when the hunter calls "In the Name of God" while shooting (Shaaranni 1999). If these conditions are not met, eating the flesh of that animal which is considered non-*halal* meat is forbidden (*haram*). Animals must be slaughtered using sharp tools towards the direction of Mecca (Qiblah) in Saudi Arabia when the slaughterer calls the name of God. (Kulayni 1987, 233–5). The issue of calling God's name while slaughtering animal is emphasized in the Qur'an (6:118). It is one of the Islamic laws (*hokm*) which demonstrates the extent of Islam's attention to the respect of creatures' lives (Jafari Tabrizi 1999, 43). It also emphasizes that killing animals can only be done with God's permission.

In addition to physical annoyance, psychological abuse of animals is also forbidden. The relevant recommendations show that Islam considers animals to have some degree of emotions. For instance, animals must not be slaughtered in front of other animals (Horr Ameli 1989, 16). Furthermore, Imam Ali asked one of his companions to avoid separating an animal and its child during shipment. Similarly, it is suggested that an animal that is raised by an individual not be slaughtered by the same person and he should buy another animal for slaughtering (Horr Ameli 1989, 91).

In addition to making laws specific to animals, numerous examples encourage kind behavior towards animals and forbid their annoyance. For instance, a narration (*revayat*) quoted from the Prophet of Islam mentions that at *Mi'rāj* (ascension), he saw a man who was suffering for tying up a cat and letting it die by not giving it food and water. He also witnessed a prostitute who was forgiven because she fetched water from a well for a thirsty dog with difficulty and used her shoes and clothes to do so (Najafi 1984, 395). Imam Ali has said that each animal's owner has six responsibilities toward his animal: (1) he should feed the animal first upon arrival at a destination; (2) he should take it near water wherever water is available; (3) he must not hit or whip it with no reason; (4) he must not put too much burden on it; (5) he must not make it walk too much; and (6) he must not sit on the animal without any reason or while it is being milked (Qomi Sadugh 1983). The Prophet has stated that animals' waist is not your seat since some animals are better than their riders and they are more valuable to God (Ravandi Kashani 1997).

## Limitations in Using Animals

In environmental ethics, it has been argued that the notions of human-centeredness and nature's subservience to humans, which are supported in some religions, have caused the destruction of nature. However, the fundamental concepts that man is a vicegerent (*khalif'a*) of God and the wonders of nature are the sign of God (*a'yah*), remind us that nature is God's trust (*amanah*) and does not need to be tamed by us. It means that man can utilize the nature according to God's will but that unauthorized use or destruction of the environment is against God's will and a failure of our responsibility as the vicegerent of God. Nature's subservience to humans does not allow every kind of consumption and exploitation, but requires humans to appropriately utilize nature's bounty in a responsible manner. Islam emphasizes the human's central role in creation as God's servant and committed to moral constraints, rather than as unconditional governors of the universe (Javadi 2008).

Imam Ali invites people to be pious and responsible towards God's creations, lands, and animals (Nahj al-Balaghah, Sermon 167). Therefore, the faithful man will consider himself responsible towards nature since he knows that he holds God's trust (*amanah*) in his hands. Islam also encourages people to live simply and prohibits a lavish lifestyle which is the starting point of environmental degradation (Javadi 2008). With respect to using animals, Islam has put many limitations. Because animals are living creatures, they are revered and harassment or abuse is not allowed unless there is a justifiable reason. For instance, killing animals for their flesh is not permitted until it is authorized by Islamic *Shari'a*. In general, Islam and the Prophet have prohibited slaughtering animals except for feeding (Majlisi 1983, 1). Therefore, hunting for pleasure is sinful (*haraam*) as well as taking part in the hunting journey.

Quoting Prophet Muhammad, it is stated that he has forbidden killing every creature with soul and even insects such as ants which are harmless. The Prophet has also mentioned that if anyone kills a sparrow without a justifiable reason, he will be questioned on the Day of Judgment (Payandeh 2003). Therefore, we may endanger an animal's life only if we have a justifiable reason. For instance on justification is to protect or save a human life. Only if human life depends on slaughtering an animal, then it is necessary to kill an animal while taking some laws and criteria into consideration. Some of those criteria have mentioned in the discussion of animal rights in Islam.

## Using Animals in Research: National Ethical Guidelines in Islamic Countries

The following examples show how Islamic countries have regulated animal use in biomedical research based on Islamic teachings. In Iran, comprehensive ethical guidelines entitled *National Ethical Guidelines for Research on Animals* were developed by the Ministry of Health and Medical Education in 2005. These guidelines endeavor to protect animals in biomedical research. It includes four topics: animal transportation; care conditions (in cages, feeding, lights, etc.); staff training; and researchers' responsibilities (National Ethical Committee on Research 2005).

In many other Islamic countries there are codes and guidelines on working with animals that take into consideration various dimensions of animal rights, for example, the National Committee of Bioethics in Saudi Arabia has developed guidelines for working with animals (Saudi National Committee on Bioethics 2013) and the King Faisal University also has specific codes for working with laboratory animals which is consistent with international research ethics codes. It requires the researchers to obtain a license and to be knowledgeable about animal care (King Faisal University 2013).

In Egypt, the ethical codes in biomedical research at Al-Azhar Faculty of Medicine include paragraphs regarding the necessity of getting a permit for using animals in biomedical research based on the required expertise to ensure animal care (Al-Azhar University 2010). Codes of professional ethics in the Faculty of Medicine at Bennha University address animal rights and the requirement to minimize their harassment (The Faculty of Medicine, 2010–2011). The research ethics guidelines in Damietta University emphasize kindness to animals and require research to be conducted under the supervision of a university expert in working with laboratory animals (Damietta University 2016).

The United Arab Emirates University's research ethics guidelines provide specific details for maintaining animal dignity and welfare (United Arab Emirates University 2014).

In Islamic countries, guidelines on using animals in biomedical research have emphasized on the following issues:

(1) When there are substitutes for laboratory animals, animals may not be used. Therefore, from the beginning, alternatives must be sought, and only when there is no other possibility, the experiments can be performed on animals under certain conditions. For instance, the least possible number of animals must be used in the research.

(2) Meeting the physical needs of animals, including appropriate food, housing, sanitation, and medication, is required (*wajib*). This includes providing care to animals that are going to die, as well as the ones that are no longer useful.

(3) Any type and degree of physical and psychological irritation and annoyance towards animals is prohibited. Some Islamic narratives have even stated that annoying animals leads to retaliation in kind (*qisas*) (Horr Ameli 1989, 485). Psychological abuse of animals is one of the neglected issues in many research systems because researchers believe animals lack emotion and cognition. Islamic teachings however emphasize the fact that Islam regards animals to have some degree of emotion and cognition. Accordingly, no animal may be killed in front of another creature, and animals must not be separated from their offspring.

(4) Licensing farmers to raise animals for research laboratories does not seem to have any prohibitions since animals are also raised for other purposes. However, it has been recommended that the person who has raised the animal should not slaughter those animals; rather, another person should slaughter the animal.

(5) After being used in medical education or research, the animal's pain must be relieved and then cared up to the end of its life.

## Conclusion

In Islam, animals as God's creatures are worthy of respect. Human beings are responsible to care for the well-being of animals and should avoid abusing them.

Medical experimentation on animals in biomedical research is inevitable for the continuing development of new drugs, procedures, and treatments to benefit humans and help improve the quality of human life. However, to also protect animal rights and welfare, limitations on using animals in medical science should be carefully regulated.

The most important principle when using animals for medical education and research is to respect animals as creatures with consciousness and thus avoid causing harm, pain, suffering, and unjustified killing. The only justification under Islamic *Shari'a* for using animals is to save human life as human life is more valued than animal life. However, compared to animals, human belongings are less valuable and thus animal life should be given priority over inanimate objects. Based on Islamic teachings, the government is responsible to care for animal rights and to make sure that owners and people working with animals treat animals well and observe animal rights.

# References

Al-Azhar University. *Vasighat Akhlaghiyat al- Bahs al- Elmi*. [*Document of Scientific Research Ethics*]. Available at: http://medicineazhar.edu.eg/attachments/article/3706/research_ethics.pdf. [Accessed August 30, 2016].

Ali ibn Abi Talib. Undated. *Nahj al-Balaghah*. Collected by Sharif Razi. Sermon 167, Letter 25.

Ameli-Shahid Thani Zayn al-din ibn Ali. 1990. *Al-rozah-ol bahiyah, fi sharhe-al lomat-ol dameshghiah*. Qom: Davari Publishing, Vol. 5, 481–2.

Ameli-Shahid Thani Zayn al-din ibn Ali. 1993. *Masalek ol-efham ela tanghi-hel sharaeel eslam*. [*Understanding of Islamic Laws*], 1st ed. Qom: Moassese Almaaref-ol Eslamiah Publishing, Vol. 15, 383; Vol. 6, 251.

Damietta University. 2016. *Guideline of Research Ethics*. Available at: http://www1.mans.edu.eg/facscid/arabic/files.pdf. [Accessed August 30, 2016].

Esfahani-Fazel Hendi Mohammad ben Hasan. 1996. *Kashf-ol letham va al-ebham an qawaed-ol ahkam*. [*Disclosure of the Rules of Judgments*], 1st ed. Qom: Eslami Publishing, Vol. 7, 612–3.

Esfahani Majlesi-e Aval, M. T. 1994. *Saheb gharani. Sharhe faghih*. 2nd ed. Qom: Moassese Esmaeelian Publishing, Vol. 7, 403.

Esfahani Majlesi-e Aval, M. T. 1980. *Yek dooreh feghhe kamel farsi*. [*A Complete Review of the Islamic Law in Persian*], 1st ed. Qom: Moassese Farahani Publishing, 186.

Hilli Hasan bin Yusof. 1993. *Qawa'id al-ahkam fi ma'rifat-al- hilal va al- haram*. [*Rules of Judgment in the Knowledge of Halal and Haraam*], 1st ed. Qom: Qom Seminary School Press, Vol. 3, 118.

Hilli Hasan bin Yusof. 1993. *Tazkirat al Fuqaha*. [*Memories of Jurists*], 1st ed. Qom: Moassese aal al-bayt Publishing, Vol. 2, 406.

Hilli Yahya ibn Saeed. 1984. *Al- jamaa lel- Sharae*. [*The Whole of the Canons*], 1st ed. Qom: Muassasat Sayyid al-Shuhada al- Elmiyah Publishing, 91.

Holy Qur'an. 2009. 3rd ed. Qom: Osveh Press.

Horr Ameli Mohammad bin Hasan. 1989. *Wasail-al shia*. [*Shi'ite Jurisprudence*], 1st ed. Qom: Moassese aal al-bayt Publishing, Vol. 11, 508, 513, 479, 496, 485; Vol. 24, 41, 16, 91–2.

Jafari-Tabrizi, M. T. 1999. *Legal treatise*. 1st ed. Tehran: Manshurat Keramat Publishing, 43, 115.

Javadi, M. 2008. Anthropocentrism in Environmental Ethics: An Islamic View. *Maqalat wa Barrasiha* (Islamic Philosophy And Kalam), 41–90; 47–66.

King Faisal University. 2013. *Ershadat Akhlaghyat al- Bahs al- Elmi. [Ethical Guidelines in Scientific Research]*, 1st ed. Available at: https://www.kfu.edu.sa/ar/Deans/Research/Documents/. [Accessed August 30, 2016].

Kulayni-Abu Jafar Mohammad bin Yaaqub. 1987. *Al-kafi.* 4th ed. Tehran: Dar-ol Kutub al-Islamiyah Publishing, Vol. 6, 544, 233–5; Vol. 7, 396; Vol. 11, 541.

La Velle, L. B. 2002. Animal Experimentation in Biomedical Research. In: Bryant, J., La Velle, L. B. and Searle, J. (eds.). *Bioethics for Scientists.* Chichester, UK: John Wiley & Sons, Ltd., 316–7.

Majlisi, M. B. 1983. *Bihar al- Anwar.* Beirut: Alwafa Institute Publishing, Vol. 61, 177, 1

Moghimi Haji, A. 2006. Animal Rights in Islamic Jurisprudence *(fiqh). Feqh-e Ahl-e Bait Journal,* 48, 138–95.

Montazeri Najaf Abadi, H. A. 1989. *Mabani-ye feqhi-ye hokumat-e eslami* (Jurisprudential basics in Islamic government). Trans. Salavati, M. and Shakuri A. Moassese. 1st ed. Qom: Keyhan Publishing, Vol. 3, 442.

Najafi Saheb Jawaher, M. H. 1984. *Jawaher al- kalam fi sharh sharaea-al-eslam. [The View Point of Jawaher al-kalam about Islamic Laws],* 7th ed. Lebanon: Dar ehya al-torath al-arabi, Vol. 27, 111; Vol. 5, 115; Vol. 31, 394–7, 307; Vol. 28, 429.

National Committee on Bio Ethics. Undated. *Research on Animals and Plants: Use of Animals and Plants in Experiments.* Available at: http://bioethics.kacst.edu.sa/Researchers/Rules-and-regulations/Conduct-research-on-animals.aspx?lang=en-US. [Accessed August 30, 2015].

National Ethical Committee on Research. Deputy of Research. Iranian Ministry of Health and Medical Education. Undated. *Ethical Guideline of Research on Animals.* Available at: http://hbi.ir/ethics/aeeinnameh/rahnamye-akhlaghi-ekhtesasi/heivanat-azmayesh.pdf. [Accessed August 20, 2015].

Payandeh, A. 2003. *Nahj al-Fasaheh.* 4th ed. Tehran: Nashre Donyaye Danesh Publishing, 751.

Qomi Sadugh-Mohammad bin ali ben Babeveyh. 1993. *Man la yahzorohol faghih. [Book for Those Who Do Not Have Access to the Islamic Jurist],* 2nd ed. Qom: Entesharat Eslami Publishing. Vol. 2, 292–3, 287.

Qomi Sadugh-Mohammad bin ali ben Babeveyh. 1983. *Al-Khisal. [Characteristics],* 1st ed. 'Ali Akbar Ghaffari (ed.). Qom: Jami'a Mudarrisin Publishing, Vol. 1, 330.

Ravandi Kashani, F. 1997. *.Al-Navader.* Trans. Sadeghi Ardestani. 1st ed. Tehran: Kooshanpour Islamic Culture foundation Publishing, 196–7.

Shaaranni, A. 1999. *Tarjome va Sharhe Tabsarat al-Mutaallimin fi Ahkam Din.* [*Translation and Explanation of the Insight of Learners in Religious Law*], 5th ed. Tehran: Manshurat Eslamiah Publishing, Vol. 2, 625.

The Faculty of Medicine for Girls, Al-Azhar University. 2010. *Misaghe Akhlaghyat al- Mehnat* [*Codes of Professionalism*] *Al-Azhar.* Available at: http://www.fmgazhar.edu.eg/qaa.html. [Accessed August 30, 2015].

The Faculty of Medicine, Benha University. 2010–2011. *Misaghe Akhlaghyat al-Momaresat* [*Code of Ethics of Practice*]. Available at: https://www.google. com/url?sa=t&rct=j&q=&esrc=s&source=web&cd=1&cad=rja&uact=8&ved =0CB4QFjAAahUKEwiF5Pinw4zIAhVGPRoKHWvBC18&url=http%3A% 2F%2Fwww.fmed.bu.edu.eg%2Ffmed%2Fimages%2Fgwda%2Fmysaka5lak. pdf&usg=AFQjCNHYlKd-RSJjsVttWYmUG-rQq8FYgA&sig2=m0YdNLK I02jpMQk6JsBhbQ. [Accessed August 30, 2016].

Tusi Abu Jafar Mohammad bin Hasan. 1968. *Al-Mabsoot fj feghhe al-Imamye.* [*Imamiyah Jurisprudence*], 3rd ed. Tehran: Al-Maktabe al-Mortazaviyeh le-Ehyae al-Asare al-Jaafarie Publishing, Vol. 6, 47.

United Arab Emirates University. 2014. *Hemayat al-Heivanat allati tojri aliha al-abhas.* [*Protection of Animals in Research*]. Available at: https://www.uaeu. ac.ae/ar/about/policies/research_and_sponsored_projects/pol_pro-ra_13_ar. pdf html. [Accessed August 30, 2015].

# CHAPTER TEN

# Biomedical Research Ethics in the Islamic Context: Reflections on and Challenges for Islamic Bioethics

## *Mehrunisha Suleman*

## Summary

This chapter will present an overview of why it is necessary to consider biomedical research ethics from the Islamic/Muslim perspective, in settings where Muslims may form a substantial proportion of the research participants or the researchers conducting trials. It will present a brief history of the historical and contemporary relevance of research ethics within the global bioethical discourse. The chapter will then offer a summary of the debates and themes relevant to biomedical research ethics from the Islamic perspective, emphasizing that this is currently an understudied area. Finally, the chapter will briefly provide a synopsis of a larger piece of research being carried out on this area by presenting the key considerations from an empirical study that assesses how Islam and its normative sources influence ethical decision-making, within the context of biomedical research, in Malaysia and Iran. This case study of female participants and research relating to intimate and domestic partner violence is a prism through which the importance of considering an Islamic perspective in biomedical research will be viewed. Islamic ethico-legal debates relating to *wilayah*, *qiwammah*, *ta'ah* and *nushuz* will be explained in relation to women's participation in research. The chapter will conclude by reflecting on the evolving role of Islamic scholarship on debates relating to gender justice in Islam and the emerging role of female scholars. Finally the chapter will highlight the existing challenges and questions that need to be addressed, from within the Islamic bioethics discourse, for the latter discourse to be responsive to emerging ethical complexities of biomedical research.

## Introduction

Islam has generally encouraged the use of science, medicine, and biotechnology as solutions to human suffering, and therefore it is important to assess Islam's influence on local ethical decision-making (Inhorn 2003). Novel ethical dilemmas presented by recent biomedical advancements have functioned as a catalyst within the Islamic scholarly sphere, compelling religious experts into renewed and sustained discussions about these challenges and the need to find appropriate solutions. As such, it would be useful to capture the Islamic perspective on the complex questions posed by global health research. Although there is substantial literature on the influence of Islam within the clinical sphere and the need for religio-culturally competent care (Padela and Punekar 2009; Inhorn and Serour 2011; Ilkilic 2002), there has been no study on the impact of the Islamic tradition on research practice and how the role of the researcher/clinician is considered from this perspective.

Islam, in this review refers to the religion, with its normative sources the Qur'an and *Sunna* (teachings of the Prophet Muhammad). However, the textual guidance needs to be considered alongside the contextual experiences of Muslims. Their lived application of the normative sources is a substrate for the growing body of Islamic legal literature. Both the textual and lived experiences need to be considered in order to understand better how Islam influences research and how Muslims, who encounter research, apply Islamic teaching in their professional and personal lives.

## *Why study the role of Islam on biomedical research ethics?*

Islam forms the second largest religious affiliation across the world and very little study has been done to explore its role in the context of research ethics. Currently there are 1.57 billion Muslims across the globe accounting for just under a quarter of the world's population (Sachedina and Ainuddin 2004). The majority of Muslims live in the developing world and therefore can form a significant cohort of research participants as well as those who carry out the research. Studies have shown that between 2006–2010 there was a 4 percent rise in the number of drug trials conducted in the Middle East (Alahmad *et al.* 2012), which includes a substantial portion of the world that ascribes to the Islamic faith. During that period, the Middle East accounted for the largest increase in such research when compared with any other regions in the world (Alahmad *et al.* 2012). Muslim majority countries in South East Asia (SEA), such as Malaysia, Indonesia, and Brunei have also displayed a rise in biomedical research. For example, benefitting from political stability following independence from British colonial rule, Malaysia has become a key economic player in SEA (Drabble 2000) and amongst the Organisation of Islamic Cooperation (OIC) countries. With a burgeoning economy, Malaysia has been keen to conduct clinical research and also be a site for outsourced clinical trials. Malaysia has become a popular site for industry and government sponsored trials because the trial process has been found to be cheaper, with faster recruitment of participants (Gross and Hirose 2007; Glickman *et al.* 2009). Countries such as Malaysia and Egypt have also recently invested in establishing research ethics committees and guidelines.[1] For example, members of research ethics committees (RECs) in Egypt considered the development of suitable national ethics guidelines as a key priority (Sleem *et al.* 2010). It is also important to consider the role religious views and values play in defining what counts as an ethical problem and what it means to be an ethical researcher. The latter is critical to gain a deeper understanding of the moral universe of Muslim researchers or the challenges researchers may face when working with a Muslim community. Another important consideration is that, within the Muslim tradition, although the formulation of religio-ethical opinions has usually been perceived as the exclusive responsibility of religious scholars, more recently, physicians and scientists themselves have taken on this task. Studies have shown that Muslim medical and scientific experts are keen to adopt the language of Islamic theology (Ghaly 2013), and to assist in drafting Islamic legal rulings in an attempt to answer emerging religio-ethical challenges. It may be pertinent to assess the nature of this emerging multifaceted role of the Muslim physicians, scientists, and researchers as well as the impact it may have on the global health research ethics discourse.

Finally, those who participate in research, together with their families, may consider their Islamic faith important when making decisions about enrolling in trials. Such considerations may include issues relating to the Islamic conception of autonomy (Sachedina 2009); what participants, families, and the broader public consider as the benefits and harms of research; and which types of research questions and interventions are considered acceptable according to the Islamic faith. Thus there are three levels at which the role of Islam on biomedical research ethics may be considered. These include factors at the global and national level; at the level of individual researchers, doctors and other healthcare professionals; and finally, at the level of research participants either as an individual, family, or community decision-making units.

The establishment and evolution of research ethics guidelines and committees will be briefly discussed before returning to their development in the Muslim world and their link to the Islamic faith.

## An Overview of Biomedical Research Ethics

In recent years, biomedical research in Low and Middle Income Countries (LAMICs) has been expanding with important implications for the development of novel, lifesaving therapies for pandemics such as HIV (Nuffield Council on Bioethics 2002). It has also been suggested that health research conducted in LAMICs may provide a valuable source of healthcare that may otherwise be unavailable to participants, whilst also enabling capacity building in the form of infrastructure development and the training of local staff (Bhutta 2002). Biomedical advancement, however, has to be carefully monitored with sufficient oversight to ensure there is no compromise of ethical standards (Lurie and Wolfe 1997). Lessons from the Nazi experiments (Weindling 2008) illustrate the importance of guidelines and regulations to ensure participant safety and protection of the local population's interests (Emanuel *et al.* 2004). Although trials on humans can be traced back several centuries, contemporary approaches aimed at protecting human subjects started only after the atrocities seen in Germany

(Caballero 2002). Following the Second World War, surviving Nazi doctors were prosecuted for war crimes at the Nuremberg trials. The resulting military tribunal articulated the Nuremberg Code in 1947 (Annas and Grodin 2008). The code banned forced experiments in humans, setting the basis for the World Medical Association's Declaration of Helsinki a few years later in 1964. These landmark documents received general international support and led to the "universal" adoption of the principle of independent, informed consent (Emanuel *et al.* 2004). Recent work on global biomedical ethics has transformed research standards dramatically, considering not only challenges in consent procedures (Freedman 1987), but also more subtle questions relating to exploitation; the need for research to be responsive to local population needs; and the sustainability of research. This shift has occurred with the growing realization that some of the most contentious contemporary ethical controversies are not related to informed consent but rather to the ethics of appropriate risk–benefit ratios, exploitation, and the value of research to the local community (Emanuel *et al.* 2000), where the endemic socio-economic injustices also cannot be overlooked (Ijsselmuiden 2010). It is also important to note here that the field of global health research ethics faces the continuing challenge of its application within ethnographically diverse settings. Although bioethics has increasingly developed a global consciousness, some authors suggest that universal principles are not available and may never be established to successfully guide ethical decision-making irrespective of cultural or religious contexts (Ryan 2004; Chattopadhyay and De Veries 2012). Despite the variety of work that has been accomplished thus far (in deriving and applying ethical principles), there are concerns that many researchers fail to take into consideration the pertinence of religious pluralism, cultural differences, and moral diversity pervading different societies (Durante 2009). These and other authors consider it therefore necessary to re-assess existing research protocols to ascertain whether they allow for the necessary cultural diversity and therefore enhance applicability. For example, it has been suggested that one of the reasons for the outsourcing of clinical trials to countries in SEA is to avoid the rigorous oversight mechanisms present in Europe and North American countries (Yusof 2015; Garrafa *et al.* 2010). Similarly, the Middle East has been considered a popular site for research due to improving infrastructure and patient diversity in addition to fewer ethical constraints in comparison with Europe and North America (Alahmad *et al.* 2012). This increase in clinical trials in the OIC countries emphasizes the need for ensuring that these sites of clinical trials have a robust governance process to ensure that the research that is taking place is ethical. The establishment of research ethics governance systems that can successfully oversee research and its development requires both intellectual and infrastructural investment. The latter and former will ensure that research being conducted within the OIC is ethically sound, avoids exploitation and the results produced by the research are valid internationally. In a study, Muslim bioethicists have identified maintaining good clinical research practices as one of the top 10 bioethical challenges facing Muslim countries, which also lists: justice, human rights, bioethics capacity building, and bioethics committees (Bagheri 2014).

## Biomedical Research Ethics: An Omission Within Islamic Bioethics

In this section, the extent to which there is an Islamic perspective on the complex questions posed by biomedical research is discussed. Although there is a burgeoning of Islamic bioethics literature addressing emerging biomedical technologies, there is little output pertaining to the ethical challenges posed by biomedical research. A recent review highlights a stark absence of literature in English addressing the bioethical challenges of human subject research from an Islamic perspective (Suleman 2015a). A reason for this may be due to the lack of collation and translation of relevant Muslim scholarly works and discussions into English. The more likely explanation for this gap is the intellectual preoccupation of scholars who are responding to specific biotechnologies, and are yet to employ their scholarly expertise to address the broader ethical questions of biomedical research, particularly human subject research.

Despite claims that countries within the Muslim world have developed "Islamic" guidelines (Kazim 2007) for the ethical conduct of research, there has been very little study of this "Islamic" influence on ethical decision-making in such settings. Three countries within the Middle East have drafted guidelines that "claim to respect Islamic law"

(Alahmad *et al.* 2010), but the definition of "Islamic law" is unclear, as are the particulars in terms of the conduct of biomedical research.

Thus far, papers in this field include an Islamic perspective on biomedical research ethics (Afifi 2007a; 2007b); Islamic adaptations by the Islamic Organisation of Medical Sciences (IOMS 2005) of the globally recognised Council for International Organizations of Medical Sciences (CIOMS 2002) guidelines; academic blogs (Kasule 2007); and a series of papers and book chapters (Sachedina 2009). However, many of those writings mention how research ethics has been overlooked in Islamic bioethics. Although a detailed overview of the literature and guidelines pertaining to biomedical research ethics from the Islamic and Muslim context has been published (Suleman 2015a; 2015b), in the next two sections a brief summary will be presented about the challenges and research gaps within this field of study.

## A focus on autonomy and the "four principles" within Islamic bioethics

"Western" secular ethics is widely accepted as "rights-based" with a strong emphasis on individual rights and freedoms. A seminal work by Beauchamp and Childress (1979) established four principles, namely autonomy, beneficence, non-maleficence, and justice. Autonomy and in turn informed consent have become important cornerstones of biomedical research, written into ethical guidelines to prevent the repetition of historical atrocities. Many authors consider autonomy to be the most important ethical principle (Engelhardt 1986).

Studies that specifically consider Islamic perspectives on research ethics principles tend to reflect on Islamic laws and values in reference to existing "western" secular ethical principles. Autonomy, for example, is discussed by numerous authors, some of whom accept it as a principle within the Islamic tradition predating Beauchamp and Childress's work (Aksoy and Tenik 2002), and agreeing with the latter authors' claim that autonomy is a universal principle shared and applied by different religio-cultural traditions. Aksoy has also explored the roots of all four principles from within the Islamic tradition (Aksoy and Elmali 2002), arguing that these principles are "already being applied in Islamic traditional and cultural societies." However, many other authors argue that although Muslims may broadly share the four principles, they differ on how these are applied within the research context. For example, autonomy and the duty to obtain a patient's informed consent are contentious issues within Islamic ethics. In Islam, the emphasis is on the individual's duty to God, to the community, and to himself. The principle of autonomy does not allow infringement of another individual's rights, unless absolutely necessary, and must be justified by the need to balance against other important duties such as preserving life and avoiding harm. In Islam an individual's freedom may be constrained if it causes harm to others (Rathor *et al.* 2011). Defining harm may be based on the principle of public good (*maslaha*) where the risk–benefit ratio is used to ascertain whether a decision would be in the public's benefit, overall.

Another important concept in Islam and within Muslim communities is the sacred position of the family (Shabana 2013). Thus, Muslims may not share the "western" secular construct of autonomy and may prefer "collective autonomy" where healthcare and health research decisions are made not only by the individual, but the entire family unit. In some Muslim societies, this decision-making process may even include religious leaders and friends (Oguz 2003). The decision-making unit, or a group (*jama'ah*), is favoured in Islam over an individual's decision. This does not mean that an individual's view is not respected, but it allows familial and community advice when making a decision and thereby retaining their support through a favourable or unfavourable outcome.

The literature review (Suleman 2015a) reveals that there is little material in English where Islamic legal thought is applied independently of existing guidelines, where many authors have simply sought the "Islamic equivalents" of the four principles. It could be argued that there is little need for additional frameworks if those that exist allow researchers to answer emerging ethical questions (ten Have and Gordijn 2011), but it may be more valuable to derive principles from within the Islamic tradition rather than trying to superimpose "western" secular ethics onto an Islamic ethico-legal framework. It has been contended, however, that there is a "western bias" within contemporary mainstream bioethics (Chattopadhyay and De Veries 2013), which can also be observed within the field of research ethics. As existing guidelines and principles have failed to enable us to overcome the injustices noted above, contributions from other traditions such as Islam may provide fresh insight into the definition of existing values, how these ought to be applied, and how those responsible should be held accountable.

One may consider that the intellectual interaction of different moral worlds and traditions is both necessary and inevitable. Many Muslim health practitioners and researchers train in the West and therefore become familiar with "western" medicine and "western" secular ethical principles. When practicing in the West or in Muslim contexts they may adapt these principles based on their environment or personal beliefs. It may not be possible for them to divorce their intellectual and professional training from Islamic pronouncements of what is ethical. Rather what may be necessary is a platform to discuss such intellectual and practical interactions to enable Muslims to remain cognisant of their training whilst having the ethico-legal and moral resources to navigate through problems that are not in harmony with their beliefs.

In order to explore these concepts and challenges in more detail, we will now focus on the ethical challenges encountered by researchers and guideline developers when considering the enrolment of Muslim women into research studies. The case study of female participants and research relating to intimate and domestic partner violence is a prism through which to view the challenges associated with, and the importance of considering, an Islamic perspective in biomedical research. The case study reveals the challenges of ensuring fairness; participants' freedom to enrol into trials; and safeguarding participants' safety and confidentiality. The following sections also outline the ethical dilemmas faced by researchers in balancing the aforementioned responsibilities while meeting the expectations of professional (national and international) guidelines, and simultaneously considering the religious and cultural environment in which they work. Researchers may, therefore, face harm due to the anxiety and moral distress that may result from the conflicting values and ideals they encounter. Finally, it is also important to glean from the following sections the harms that may result if women are excluded from biomedical research and/or encounter barriers to participation that cause them to refrain from taking part in research studies. Such barriers can lead to harms to scientific knowledge, harms to female participants who are unable to participate in trials that matter to them, and their health, and the health of other women.

## Biomedical Research Ethics in the Islamic Context: The Status and Role of Female Participants

Within the discussion around the Islamic perspective on research ethics lies the question and controversy of female consent. The status of women is a commonly disputed area within Islam. Although spiritually equal to men, where the Qur'an emphasises this spiritual equality, (16:97), physically, women are offered the protection of men through their fathers, guardians, or husbands (4:34). This Qur'anic principle is taken to imply that women are more vulnerable and therefore need protection, and the application of the latter principle often leads to discordance within the Muslim community. For example, in research settings, some authors suggest that a married woman may only participate if she has first sought the permission of her husband. A husband may not, however, force his wife to participate in a trial (Afifi 2007b). Seeing it as a religious duty, with such interpretation originating from the Qur'an, women may consider their husband's permission as imperative, and such a decision may be described as exercising her second order autonomy rights (Keyserlingk 1993). Others have, however, argued that it is not in accordance with a woman's human rights to have to seek her husband's permission before participating in a trial (Fadel 2010). The latter consensus was established by the Islamic Organisation of Medical Sciences (IOMS). However, the IOMS guideline added that "although not a requirement, it is preferable for a married woman to obtain her husband's consent" (IOMS 2005). The statement is ambiguous, however, with no details regarding the circumstances in which a husband's permission would be necessary. Another important ethical consideration is that women are often marginalized in communities and may not access healthcare. Does the suggestion of consultation with their protectors empower women to have the necessary discussions with the male members of the household where such conversations may be necessary and common, or does it cause them to withdraw further from accessing services? The ambiguity in the interpretation of the normative texts, however, reveals that more may be at play in determining gender roles in Muslim communities.

The following two sections draw on themes, questions, and challenges from an empirical investigation (Suleman 2016) that was carried out to study in more detail the issue of the status and role of women in biomedical research, within Islamic contexts, particularly relating to research pertaining to domestic and intimate partner violence.

### *The role and status of female participants in research: What we learn from empirical data*

Within a detailed study of biomedical research ethics in the Islamic context (Suleman 2016) the literature and guideline review (Suleman 2015a; 2015b; 2016), revealed that, although international guidelines have been adapted to incorporate Islamic views, studies have shown that they are of limited practical application within a "Muslim country" setting (Sleem *et al.* 2010). An empirical study was carried out in two case study sites to assess the extent to which Islam influences ethical decision-making within the context of biomedical research. Fifty-six semi-structured interviews were carried out in Malaysia (38) and Iran (18) with researchers, REC members, guideline developers, and Islamic scholars to understand whether Islam influences what they consider to be an ethico-legal problem, and how such issues are addressed. The detailed methods and results of the study can be found in the original thesis that will be published in due course (Suleman 2016), however, a summary of some of the themes and questions emerging from the empirical study, evaluated through a framework analysis (Lewis and Rithchie 2003, 56), will be presented here. This and subsequent sections explore whether Muslim communities require women to seek permission and whether it is the religious texts that influence these social norms. Although, male and female researchers were interviewed, male and female research participants were not, the collection of such empirical data may be the focus of future work in this area.

The research ethics guidelines in Malaysia[2] and Iran (Zahedi and Larijani 2008; Larijani *et al.* 2005) do not cite IOMS nor do they mention any religious or cultural consideration of seeking permission and/or co-consent, where the man (husband, father, or guardian) has consented alongside the woman. During the discussions with participants, however, it became clear that researchers and RECs struggled with the issue of co-consent or the need for women to seek permission and would have appreciated assistance from guidelines. Each of the participants in Malaysia and Iran were asked about their views and experience of enrolling female participants. Although very few were aware of IOMS, many did consider the religious and/or cultural role of women and men and cited either the Qur'an or sayings of the Prophet to explain their viewpoint. For example, one of the participants in Malaysia explained in relation to informed consent, "if you were to go strict with the Islamic paradigm, the wife has got to get the permission of the husband, that's the Islamic concept."[3] Participants, however, explained that they considered an ethical distinction between providing women the necessary clinical care where no such permission is needed versus access or enrolment into research studies, which are not necessary to maintain health. A respondent explained that "for research I don't mind (using this paradigm) but for something that is established, medical fact, our ruling or our stand in the hospital is that the wife can actually forego the husband's objection."[4] His view suggests that as medical treatment has an established benefit, then a husband should not be able to influence access to such care. However, as research may not confer such benefit and may involve greater risks, then the husband's role as guardian ought to be considered and/or respected.

This senior researcher further explained that although he might personally disagree with the husband's view, he felt obligated to respect this religo-cultural dimension of authority within a marital relationship. He presented his experience and understanding of Islam where the husband is considered the "protector" of the wife and is, therefore, given overall responsibility within a marital relationship. He did, however, explain that in instances where a medical intervention is considered of specific benefit to the wife, the *Sharia* council may override the husband's view in order to protect the rights of the woman. Yet, medical research is exploratory and unless it is considered to be of benefit to the woman's life, then according to his view, a husband is considered to have the right to be asked, and to then be able to refuse his wife's participation. Again, he did consider, however, that a husband's ability to influence or deter his wife from carrying out an altruistic act might not be something he would agree with but would need to respect. The researcher also reflected on a very important consideration, which is that the verse of the Qur'an he relies upon for developing and maintaining such an understanding of gender roles and subsequently his responsibility in such contexts, "has been interpreted in many different ways." These differing interpretations and participants' views will be explored in more detail in the next sections along with the impact of conservative interpretations on the views of RECs and their consideration of research proposals relating to women's health.

In Malaysia, respondents explained that despite such views about their deferring authority to husbands/male guardians in the enrolment of women in research, amongst researchers, REC members, and guideline developers, the guidelines do not stipulate a requirement for consulting the husband nor do they emphasize clearly that such a consideration is unnecessary. One of the guideline developers explained that the guidelines were deliberately silent on the issue to allow researchers, participants, and their families to decide for themselves. Also, it was mentioned that as Malaysia has a national strategic interest in attracting overseas researchers and funders, the guidelines that were developed were kept non-specific.

In Iran, by contrast, the participants explained that the issue of female consent was systematically considered when drafting the research ethics guidelines and involved formal consultation with scholars. Unless the research pertained to issues "relating to the family" co-consent/co-consultation was not necessary. It is important to mention here that in both Malaysia and Iran, participants (both male and female) referenced the notion that a husband's permission is necessary for a wife to leave her house. The normative textual origins of this and the interpretations of the latter in different geographical and cultural contexts will be explored in the next section.

Many participants in Malaysia and Iran explained that the husband's view would be necessary if the wife's participation affected the marriage. Effects on the marriage included:

- Excessive time spent away from home (away from children, household commitments);
- Accepting researchers into the home. This was considered problematic as the house in Muslim families in Malaysia and Iran is often

owned by the husband, and there may be concerns about gossip (*fitnah*) if the wife was seen to be accepting male visitors without the husband's knowledge. Some cited the authentic narration of the Prophet where he advised that a wife should not accept visitors without her husband's permission (*Sahih Bukahri,* Book 18, *Hadith* 1750);

- If the research had the potential to affect the wife's fertility/sexual function;
- If the potential participant was pregnant;
- If the research concerned medical interventions that required the husband's permission, e.g. abortion, contraception, sterilization;
- If the wife/participant herself considered the husband's permission necessary.

Although the enforcement of such a recommendation may be challenging and variable, it is important to note the difference in approaches between Malaysia and Iran. As there is a centralised consideration of Islamic values in Iran, the guideline developers considered it necessary to initiate a consultation on the issue of female consent and arrived at a pragmatic conclusion that was considered acceptable according to international expectations of ethical standards as well as local religious considerations. In Malaysia, however, although some researchers also expressed a similar pragmatism and concern for the family, rather than a strict distinction between a man and a woman's consent, there were researchers who had experienced uncertainty and stated that in situations where they had attempted to enrol a woman into a trial and the husband disagreed, they did not pursue her enrolment.

There were other researchers, in Malaysia and Iran, many of whom were women, who contested the co-consent/permission view and considered that the guidelines ought to be followed as they had been written and that the issue of co-consent/permission was cultural and had been religiously endorsed through particular interpretations of Islamic normative sources. Many of the researchers considered a pragmatic approach in situations where they were keen to accommodate a woman's belief and concern for consulting her husband; or followed the deferral model if the husband expressed a strong opinion; or allowed time for husband/family consultation if the researcher him/herself considered it appropriate. At the same time there were other researchers and REC members who were critical of this approach. They disagreed with this conservative view of women's autonomy. Many expressed frustration at there being a lack of adherence to the more progressive guidelines. Some also mentioned an important observation in Malaysia that the issue of co-consent or deferral to the husband was not primarily a religious concern as it was also encountered with non-Muslim participants. Participants in Malaysia explained that this impression regarding the role and status of women was due to the cultural influence, which had permeated into a religious narrative. These challenges will be explored further in the next section.

## The concepts of wilayah and qiwamah in the context of research

This section will review the Qur'anic terms and concepts of *wilayah* (guardianship of men over women) and *qiwamah* (a degree of strength or authority that is afforded to men over women) within the biomedical research ethics context. The above section highlights how the religious and cultural impressions of the role of men and women became important to participants. In terms of the religious context, participants offered verses of the Qur'an or sayings of the Prophet as explanations for their views. It became clear during the discussions that a deeper exploration of these views and interpretations was necessary in order to understand whether it was the Islamic normative sources that were informing such views or whether cultural influences inspired these particular interpretations of these sources. One of the participants in Iran expressed very strong views about consent and autonomy in Muslim societies and what he articulated as an Islamic perspective, rooted in the normative sources of Islam. He explained that the Islamic tradition does not focus on the individual but on their relationship with God. Decision-making also is not focused on the individual but the family. He explained that when two people, a man and a woman, come together to create a family, their role and their autonomy is different from when they were single: "Autonomy of man and woman unmarried is different of autonomy of man and woman that married. Autonomy of mine before I married my wife is different to after I was married. I have lower autonomy after I got married.

My autonomy is lower because I accept my job in my family."[5] He explained that in Islam the role of family is more important than the individuals within it. However, the family itself requires a lead and "that Islam gives man superiority for management of family. It does not mean that man is better than woman."[6]

This characterisation of autonomy is distinct to the description in, for example, Beauchamp and Childress's seminal work on biomedical ethics (Beauchamp and Childress 2001). Although the previous participant's description seems to point to both men and women having equal responsibility and freedom to serve the needs of their family, he highlights that according to his understanding of the Qur'an, the man has been given "superiority" and therefore may exercise the power to set the agenda for what is in the family's best interests.

Other participants described that there are problems with such a view, including the supposition that the man can decide what these "best interests" are without unduly placing his needs above the needs of his wife and family. Respondents explained that there may be a conflict of interest which causes problems including the wife's inability to act altruistically when that is her preferred choice and would confer her the benefit of having contributed to medical knowledge. Her husband may, however, intervene and prevent her enrolment arguing for her safety but is in fact more concerned for his own convenience such as ensuring he does not have to unduly take on more responsibility of the children or housework. Researchers explained that disentangling such motivations might be incredibly complex and unachievable.

Others, including Islamic scholars in both Malaysia and Iran, contested this interpretation of guardianship (*wilayah*) and authority (*qiwamah*) as being the result of patriarchal interpretations of the Qur'an, where Islamic scholarship and especially the translation and exegesis of the Qur'an have been male dominated. One male Islamic scholar in Malaysia explained that such interpretations have prevailed as: "commentators on the Qur'an (*mufasirun*) are mostly Muslim men." Some of the participants stressed the importance of looking at different environments to understand why particular interpretations of Islam are adopted. Several participants in Iran mentioned that the Iranian understanding of the role and status of women was distinct to that in other parts of the Muslim world, particularly the

Arab states. One author who studied Muslim family law in Arab countries analysed what is commonly considered to be "patriarchal religiously-justified laws in Muslim countries" (Al Hibri 1997, 2). Her study looked at the personal status codes of: Egypt, Algeria, Morocco, Tunisia, Syria, Jordan, and Kuwait. Until recently, all of these countries listed or implied "a duty of obedience (ta'ah) by the wife" (Al Hibri 1997, 11).

Political changes in Tunisia have brought family law reforms that have replaced such an "obedience" clause with the man simply being described as the head of the family (Al Hibri 1997, 11). These codes are important as they specify that obedience precludes a wife's ability to leave the husband's house without his permission. And if she were to leave without permission she would be deemed sinful, disobedient (nushuz), and no longer eligible for financial support (Al Hibri 1997, 12). Such constructions of Islamic law and interpretations of scripture, though formed in Arab states, have influenced learning and understanding in other countries. Although women occupy the highest positions in office in both Malaysia and Iran, there is a lack of clarity about the "Islamic" understanding of the role and status of women, particularly within the family. Many of the participants, including scholars, explained that the verses mentioning wilayah, qiwamah, and nushuz were commonly interpreted and applied in isolation of the broader message of the Qur'an which emphasises equality between men and women.

Some of the participants, including Islamic scholars, explained that Islam, through its ability to influence behaviour and wield political or social power, is used to accentuate a particular culture. Islamic jurisprudence enables the use of culture (urf) to set religious norms and individual reason (ijtihad) by scholars to emphasise particular values and principles. In the predominantly patriarchal societies that have prevailed in Muslim societies, it is unsurprising therefore to encounter patriarchal reasoning and culture influencing Islamic jurisprudence where scholars have interpreted religious texts to derive laws related to their cultural milieu (Al Hibri 1997, 42). The cultural environment of scholars can therefore lead to a permissive or restrictive interpretation. Historically for women, because their lives and concerns fall within traditional structures of power and authority, these environments led to religious scripture legitimising/accentuating cultural practices that then became inter-generational practices, open to diminishing scrutiny due to the established legal precedent (Ramadan 2009).

Some of the participants in Malaysia explained that it is necessary to constantly survey the laws of Islam and re-examine religious interpretation and jurisprudence to ensure the rights of women and men and the interests of society are met given the evolving local and global contexts and cultures. Participants also highlighted that it is not the religious texts that influence these social norms; rather, it is the cultural traditions independent of religion shared by other faith communities in the region that impact the interpretation of the texts. In the light of participants' views relating to the sensitivity of Qur'anic interpretation, it is important to briefly consider the factors that influence exegesis. Authors who have written on this subject state that there are at least four factors to consider (Von Denffer 1983, 41–42):

— The semantics or what is said within the text, and whether the text itself can be an explanation — the synchronic significance of scriptural interpretation;
— Consideration of a verse/text within the whole revelation and the whole period of revelation — the diachronic significance of scriptural interpretation (Ramadan 2009);
— When the semantics are open, it is important to consider the cultural projection or the environment of revelation, including the tradition of the Prophet;
— The interpretation of the text through the tradition of scholars, e.g. each of the four/five schools of Islamic law may have their own rules of Qur'anic interpretation.

Thus far, for the interpretation of the word *qawwamun*, the "superiority" of men over women, has been most commonly used, followed by "having authority over", and finally, the least common opinion is "taking care of" (Mir Hosseini *et al.* 2015). Some authors have even suggested that it may even be considered "men are the servants of women" (El Fadl 2014). The last two interpretations emphasize that the man has the duty to take care of the family and the woman has the right not to work and be looked after. However, the cultural handling of the interpretations reveals that scholars have preferred the first interpretation as they have lived in and experienced only patriarchal societies. Their contextual reality informs them that men have a status superior to women so when they read the text they consider it as confirming this view. However, recent discussions and debates amongst those calling for a reform in how the Qur'an is interpreted are proposing that scholars should take the text and challenge the context, rather than use the text to justify their context (Ramadan 2009, 207–32).

Scholars have considered such verses as ambiguous (El Fadl 2014) in comparison to those relating to the more ritualistic practices of Islam where God's command is clear. This distinction is important in the context of biomedical research ethics as a balance must be drawn between respecting local cultures (Chattopadhyay and De Veries 2012), and inadvertently breaching ethical standards (Macklin 1999). Many of the participants in Iran and Malaysia mentioned the importance of raising public awareness and public debate regarding research ethics issues to ensure the concerns within the professional sphere are not raised in isolation but address the needs of the public. Their experience highlighted the difference in awareness and understanding between the public and professional spheres relating to religious interpretation and scripture. The following section sets out in more detail these concerns relating to the religious interpretations of normative texts.

## Challenges in Research on Intimate and Domestic Partner Violence

The World Health Organization (WHO) has reported: "violence against women by an intimate partner is a major contributor to the ill-health of women" (Garcia-Moreno *et al.* 2006). Views expressed by participants revealed that research on intimate and domestic partner violence was challenging in Muslim contexts, beyond the oft-described issues of privacy, confidentiality, safety, and participant vulnerability (Ellsberg *et al.* 2001). Participants explained that what is considered domestic violence is contextually dependent. Some participants explained that due to the acceptance of *wilayat* in Muslim households, where the man is considered the guardian or superior, there is a different understanding of "domestic violence." Of course, contextual adaptations and translations of such terms are necessary; however, some participants expressed reluctance to conduct or approve such research. One female researcher in Iran, however, explained that such concerns had little to do with Islam or scriptural interpretation, and had more to do with cultural influences and husbands feeling threatened by such research. She explained that: "in our country, based on our cultural issues, it's very difficult to ask women about domestic violence ... those who are governing that province says, 'stop that research, that you're not allowed to do this research in our province because of the cultural issues we have, you're not allowed.'"[7]

There was an appreciable sensitivity about such research as the men felt threatened that their wives would demand a different relationship and different freedoms. Although in Iran there are less conservative views about a wife's ability to freely leave her home, decide whom she meets and whom she invites home, the above quote reflects that there is an underlying concern/influence that resembles the patriarchy observed in other Muslim countries, such as the Arab states (Al Hibri 1997, 2). The WHO study on intimate partner violence stated that it is particularly difficult to study and respond effectively to such violence as many women and societies accept such violence as "normal." When researchers were asked about such concerns, they explained that one particular verse of the Qur'an, that states:

Men are in charge of women by [right of] what Allah has given one over the other and what they spend [for maintenance] from their wealth. So righteous women are devoutly obedient, guarding in [the husband's] absence what Allah would have them guard. But those [wives] from whom you fear arrogance — [first] advise them; [then if they persist], forsake them in bed; and [finally], strike them. But if they obey you [once more], seek no means against them. Indeed, Allah is ever Exalted and Grand (4:34).

This verse has been interpreted, accepted, and applied within Muslim societies, and has not only justified such violence but has caused Muslim women to feel that they must accept such treatment as belonging within the fold of Islam and that they are deserving of such violence because of their own behaviour. One researcher in Malaysia who has done extensive work on women's health explained that researching intimate partner violence is particularly challenging because: "when you talk about values, for example, it's very difficult for people, for survivors of domestic violence, to actually just disconnect with their husband because they think that religion gives a certain interpretation about men and wives relationship."[8] She explained that: "when you want to engage them on this dialogue about what obedience is all about, you're really trying to intrude into their faiths sometimes because you're trying to get them to have this dialogue with you ... do we start this dialogue with them or not? If I don't do it, at the back of my mind, as a believer, and I want to give them information, who can give this information, and what kind of information, that they should have so that they can process this whole idea about this rules that they have in mind about obedience, so that they can be really knowledgeable, so that they can make the right decision?"[9] The researcher's experience reveals a deep ethical challenge where, as a Muslim herself, she feels it is important to represent her faith but is concerned about the scientific requirements of the study and also the ethical and welfare implications of her intervention. It is important to point out here her emphasis on the trend discovered in her research which reveals how many religions, not only Islam, have particular ideas about "obedience" of the wife within marriage. Such a trend again points to particular cultural views and practices that are then accentuated by patriarchal religious interpretations.

Her experience highlights some key challenges in ensuring that such research can be carried out, accepted, and can lead to necessary health systems and policy changes. She explained further that the so-called religious objection to the promotion of women's rights is on the basis that such views are un-Islamic or "western" secular, and that such secularisation ought to be challenged. This narrow view of Islam and Islamic ethics ought to be confronted by scholars and political leaders as well as health providers and researchers. A public debate about such issues will enable the collation and addressing of such concerns whilst promoting public education. One Islamic scholar also suggested that such views exist and remain within societies because of women's lack of economic freedom. Many scholars have commented that Islam was recognised during its advent and early years as being a religious revolution in providing women unprecedented financial freedom through their being able to inherit wealth and own property (Kung 2007, 562). Fazlur Rahman, the distinguished

Islamic scholar, has been noted to have reflected that "in its initial phase, Islam was moved by a deep rational and moral concern for reforming society, and that this moral intentionality was conceived in ways that encouraged a deep commitment to reasoning and rational discourse" (Nanji 1993, 107).

Some authors have suggested verse 4:34 ought to be interpreted based on domestic arrangements and capacities. If the wife is the breadwinner then she is the one entrusted with the "burden of guardianship" (El Fadl 2014). Additionally, such a verse cannot be interpreted in isolation of other verses of the Qur'an and also the narrations of the Prophet (El Fadl 2001). The Prophet stated that: "The best of you is the one who is best to his wife" (Ibn Majah, Vol. 3, Book 9, *Hadith* 1977), nor did he ever beat his wife (Ibn Majah, Vol. 3, Book 9, *Hadith* 1984). As explained above, the example of the Prophet is a key factor when interpreting the Qur'an, so the neglect of such authentic narrations of *hadith* in the interpretation of verse 4:34 must be re-examined. A recent re-examination of such Qur'anic verses, from a woman's perspective, whilst referring to the pre-existing tradition (Wadud 1999, 74–6), explains that the terms *nushuz* cannot mean "disobedience to the husband" as it refers to both the man and the woman, and is more likely to refer to "marital disharmony." Wadud's seminal work suggests that "*daraba*" does not mean "to hit", rather it can mean "to set as an example" or "to leave" (Wadud 1999, 74–6). Overall, she suggests that the Qur'an is pointing to methods of dealing with marital disharmony rather than pointing individually to the man or woman. More importantly, the Qur'anic verse does not condone violence against women which supports the overall spirit of the Qur'an and therefore, as explained above, would not contradict accepted methods of Qur'anic interpretation. Wadud explains clearly that the problem of domestic violence in Muslim families is "not rooted in this Qur'anic passage." She explains that the men who hit their wives are not seeking marital harmony, rather are simply motivated to harm them (Wadud 1999, 74–6). Wadud's work and that of other scholars such as Khaled Aboul Fadl (El Fadl 2001), suggest that the message of Islam is clear, and it is convenient for certain structures of power and authority to promote and retain particular interpretations of the normative sources to bolster their own cultural preferences.

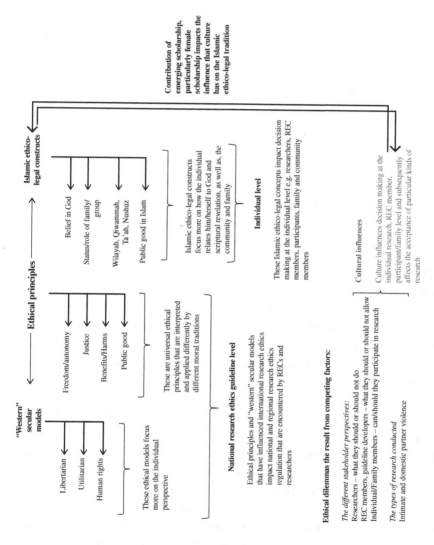

**Figure 1:**   Factors and influences encountered by researchers in Islamic contexts.

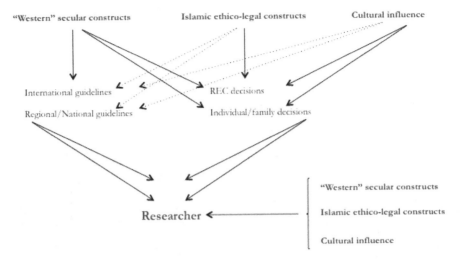

**Figure 2:**   Researchers have to grapple with different ethico-legal, cultural and moral traditions.

The above diagrams illustrate the many factors and influences encountered by researchers in Islamic contexts. They demonstrate the different facets when considering the principles of freedom/autonomy, justice, benefits/harms and public good, in relation to the participation of women in research. The diagrams highlight the interaction, overlap, and complexity involving "western" secular constructs, the Islamic ethico-legal discourse, and cultural perspectives.

These competing pressures highlight that researchers may encounter ethico-legal challenges that are presented as being from within the Islamic tradition, but are in fact only considered so *post hoc* due to cultural influences. Although national guidelines may not stipulate co-consent and uphold international standards, there is a complex interplay of culture, religion, and other moral sources at the level of RECs, participants, and families. Researchers must therefore grapple with such complex factors, as well as their own individual moral leanings to come to a decision about what they ought to do when considering research pertaining to women. These factors seem to also suggest that the role of the Islamic ethico-legal tradition in biomedical research ethics can be to redress the balance of freedom, justice, safety, and benefit for women that may have been under-mined by cultural pressures. Islam and Islamic scholarship can therefore make a critical contribution by helping to address the ambiguity and con-tentions related to the role and status of women that can enable REC mem-bers/researchers/families/participants to come to a decision that is cognizant of their faith while still upholding the broader ethical standards.

## Conclusions

This chapter has attempted to emphasize that research ethics is a nascent field and must be fully incorporated within the field of Islamic bioethics. Those who are engaging in the Islamic bioethical discourse have a unique opportunity to contribute to evolving global thought on research ethics. They can join efforts with a plethora of specialists already at the table, including anthropologists, philosophers, theologians, social scientists, health professionals as well as those versed in spirituality and psychology. Failing to engage promptly will find Islamic bioethicists playing intellec-tual catch-up or simply negotiating terminology without participating in the thought-shift about ethico-legal questions and solutions relating to human subject research in the Islamic context. They have a key role in contributing to discussions around the issue of women's status and role in biomedical research. Although some countries like Iran have provided clear guidance with the assistance of Islamic scholars on this issue, many other countries that have a significant Muslim population may have researchers who continue to be faced with ambiguity and anxiety about how to appropriately approach and enrol female participants, as well as how to protect the welfare of the participants. The synopsis of the empiri-cal study presented here highlights the contested interpretation of reli-gious scripture regarding the role and status of women in biomedical research. In the professional sphere, there are on-going scholarly discus-sions at the state level in Iran emphasising equal roles and rights of women and men individually and in the family. In Malaysia, as Islam is not organised at the national level and the guidelines are silent, research-ers and REC members are left to decide for themselves. This does, how-ever, raise the issue of how conservative interpretations of religious scripture affect not only the professional sphere but also the public sphere.

Yet Islam's underlying flexibility means that after centuries of disengagement from the texts and scholarly discourse, Muslim women are reclaiming their seat within Islamic scholarship and not only calling for a re-examination but also rereading the sacred texts for themselves. The discussion does not suggest a monoculture within Muslim societies, rather a predominant view within the laity that emphasises male superiority within the family. One of the foremost scholars of Islam, Ibn al Qayyim Al Jawziyyah stated that: "The purpose of God's way is the establishment of righteousness and justice … so any road that establishes what is right and just is the road (Muslims) should follow" (Grote and Tilmann 2011, 42). Although recent Muslim societies have seen a predominance of male scholarship and patriarchal interpretations, there is an increasing voice amongst scholars and professionals providing contextual and textual challenges to the *status quo*. The future of Islamic ethics is reliant on such scholarly flexibility and this dynamism is likely to lead to positive ethical approaches to the inherently difficult biomedical/bioethical problems described and which include: the potential harms that may result from the exclusion of women and pregnant women from biomedical research, including harm to scientific knowledge; harm to female participants who are unable to participate in trials that matter to them and their health and the health of women; and harm to researchers due to the anxiety and moral distress that may result from encountering conflicting values and ideals.

## Notes

1   Malaysia Medical Research and Ethics Committee (MREC). http://nih.gov. my/web/mrec/ [Accessed on 18 May 2016].
2   http://www.nccr.gov.my/view_file.cfm?fileid=16 [Accessed on 18 May 2016].
3,4   Malaysia Interview 21, Researcher, REC member, guideline developer.
5   Iran Interview 11, Researcher, REC member.
6   Iran Interview 11, Researcher, REC member.
7   Iran Interview 13, Researcher, REC member, guideline developer.
8   Malaysia Interview 25, Researcher, REC member.
9   Malaysia Interview 25, Researcher, REC member.

## References

Ad Hoc Committee on Health Research Relating to Future Intervention Options. 1996. *Investing in Health Research and Development*. Geneva: World Health Organization.

Afifi, Raafat Y. 2007a. Biomedical Research Ethics: An Islamic View, Part II. *International Journal of Surgery* (5)6, 381–3.

Afifi, Raafat Y. 2007b. Biomedical Research Ethics: An Islamic View, Part I. *International Journal of Surgery* 5(5), 292–6.

Aimi Yusof. 2015. *Ethical Issues in Research Ethics Governance and Their Application to the Malaysian Context*. DPhil thesis. Oxford: University of Oxford.

Aksoy S. and Elmali A. 2002. Four Principles of Bioethics as found in Islamic Tradition. *Medicine and Law Journal* 21, 211–24.

Aksoy, S. and Tenik, A. 2002. The Four Principles of Bioethics as Found in 13th Century Muslim Scholar Mawlana's Teachings. *BMC Medical Ethics* 3(1), 4.

Al-Hibri, Azizah. 1997. Islam, Law And Custom: Redefining Muslim Women's Rights. *American University International Law Review* 12(1), 1–44.

Alahmad, G., Mohammad Al-Jumah and Dierickx, K. 2012. Review of National Research Ethics Regulations and Guidelines in Middle Eastern Arab Countries. *BMC Medical Ethics* 13(1), 34.

Amina Wadud. 1999. *Qur'an and Woman Rereading the Sacred Text from a Woman's Perspective*. 2nd ed. New York, Oxford: Oxford University Press.

Annas, G. and Grodin, M. The Nuremberg Code. In: Emanuel, E., Grady, C., Crouch, R., Lie, R., Miller, F. and Wendler, D. (eds.). 2008. *The Oxford Textbook of Clinical Research Ethics*. New York: Oxford University Press, 136–40.

Baker, R. W. 2015. *One Islam, Many Muslim Worlds: Spirituality, Identity, and Resistance Across Islamic Lands*. New York: Oxford University Press.

Bagheri, A. 2014. Priority Setting in Islamic Bioethics: Top 10 Bioethical Challenges in Islamic Countries. *Asian Bioethics Review* 6(4), 391–401.

Beauchamp, T. L. and Childress, J. F. 1979. *Principles of Biomedical Ethics*. New York: Oxford University Press.

Berlinguer, G. 2004. Bioethics, Health, and Inequality. *Lancet* 364(9439), 1086–91.

Bhutta, Z. 2002. Ethics in International Health Research: A Perspective from the Developing World. *Bulletin of the World Health Organization* 80(2), 114–20.

Caballero, B. 2002. Ethical Issues for Collaborative Research in Developing Countries. *American Journal of Clinical Nutrition* 76(4), 717–20.

Chattopadhyay, S. and De Veries, R. 2012. Respect for Cultural Diversity in Bioethics is an Ethical Imperative. *Medicine, Health Care and Philosophy* 16(4), 639–45.

Council on Health Research for Development (COHRED). 2000. *International Conference on Health Research for Development, Bangkok.* Available at: www.conference2000.ch.

Curran, W. J. 1973. Law-Medicine Notes: The Tuskegee Syphilis Study. *NEJM* 289, 730–1.

Drabble, H. John. 2000. *An Economic History of Malaysia, c.1800–1990: The Transition To Modern Economic Growth.* Basingstoke: Macmillan.

Durante, C. 2009. Bioethics in a Pluralistic Society: Bioethical Methodology in Lieu of Moral Diversity. *Medicine, Health Care and Philosophy* 12, 35–47.

El Fadl, K. A. 2014. *Speaking in God's Name: Islamic Law, Authority and Women.* London: Oneworld Publications.

El Fadl, K. A. 2001. The Search for Beauty in Islam: A Conference of the Books. Lanham, MD: Rowman and Littlefield.

Ellsberg, M, *et al.* 2001. Researching Domestic Violence Against Women: Methodological and Ethical Considerations. *Studies in Family Planning* 32, 1–16.

Emanuel, E., Wendler, D. and Grady, C. 2000. What Makes Clinical Research Ethical? *Journal of the American Medical Association* 283(20), 2701–11.

Emanuel, E., Wendler, D., Killen, J. and Grady, C. 2004. What Makes Clinical Research in Developing Countries Ethical? The Benchmarks of Ethical Research. *Journal of Infectious Diseases* 189, 930–7.

Engelhardt, H. T. 1986. *The Foundations of Bioethics.* Oxford; New York: Oxford University Press.

Fadel, H. E. 2010. Ethics of Clinical Research: An Islamic Perspective. *Journal of the Islamic Medical Association of North America* 42(2), 59–69.

Freedman, B. 1987. Scientific Value and Validity as Ethical Requirements for Research. *IRB:Ethics and Human Research* 9, 7–10.

Frieden, T. R., Collins, F. S. 2010. Intentional Infection of Vulnerable Populations in 1946–1948: Another Tragic History Lesson. *Journal of the American Medical Association* 304(18), 2063–4.

Garcia-Moreno, C., *et al.* 2006. Prevalence of Intimate Partner Violence: Findings from the WHO Multi-Country Study on Women's Health and Domestic Violence. *Lancet* 368(9543), 1260–9.

Garrafa, V., Solbakk, J. H., Vidal, S. and Lorenzo C. 2010. Between the Needy and the Greedy: The Quest for a Just and Fair Ethics of Clinical Research. *Journal of Medical Ethics* 36, 500–4.

Ghaly, M. 2013. Collective Religio Scientific Discussions on Islam and HIV/AIDS: I. Biomedical Scientists. *Zygon* 48(3), 671–708.

Glickman, S. W., McHutchison, J. G., Peterson, E. D., Cairns, C. B., Harrington, R. A., Califf, R. M. and Schulman, K. A. 2009. Ethical and scientific implications of the globalization of clinical research. *New England Journal of Medicine* 360(8), 816–23.

Global Forum for Health Research. 2004. *10/90 Report on Health Research 2003–2004*. Switzerland: Global Forum for Health Research.

Gross, A. and Hirose, M. 2007. *Conducting Clinical Trials in Asia*. Available at: http://www.pacificbridgemedical.com/publications/asia/2007_conducting_clinical_trials. [Accessed 4th January 2015].

Grote, R. and Roder, T. 2011. *Constitutionalism in Islamic Countries: Between Upheaval and Continuity*. Oxford: Oxford University Press, 42.

Ibn Majah. Undated. *Chapter on Marriage: "The Messenger of Allah never beat any of his servants, or wives, and his hand never hit anything."* Available at: http://sunnah.com/urn/1263030. [Accessed 2nd March 2016].

Ibn Majah. Undated. *Chapter on Marriage: "It was narrated from Ibn 'Abbas that: the Prophet said: 'The best of you is the one who is best to his wife, and I am the best of you to my wives.'"* Available at: http://sunnah.com/urn/1262960. [Accessed 2nd March 2016].

Ijsselmuiden, C. B., *et al.* 2010. Evolving Values in Ethics and Global Health Research. *Global Public Health* 5(2), 154–63.

Ilkilic, I. 2002. Bioethical Conflicts Between Muslim Patients and German Physicians and the Principles of Biomedical Ethics. *Medicine and Law* 21(2), 243–56.

Inhorn, M. C. 2003. *Local Babies, Global Science: Gender, Religion and In Vitro Fertilisation in Egypt*. New York: Routledge.

Inhorn, M. C. and Serour, G. I. 2011. Islam, Medicine, and Arab-Muslim Refugee Health in America After 9/11. *Lancet* 378(9794), 935–43.

Islamic Organization for Medical Sciences. 2005. International Ethical Guidelines for Biomedical Research Involving Human Subjects: An Islamic Perspective. In: El-Gendy, A. R., Al-Awadi, A. R. A. (eds.). *The International Islamic Code for Medical and Health Ethics, Volume 2.* Kuwait: Islamic Organization for Medical Sciences, 121–276.

Kasule, O. H. 2007. *Biomedical Research Ethics According to Islamic Law.* Available at: http://omarkasule-04.tripod.com/id1624.html. [Accessed 31st May 2015].

Katz, J., Capron, A. M. and Glass, E. S. 1972. *Experimentation with Human Beings: The Authority of the Investigator, Subject, Professions, and State in the Human Experimentation Process.* New York: Russell Sage Foundation.

Kazim, F. 2007. *Critical Analysis of the Pakistan Medical Dental Council Code and Bioethical Issues.* Master's Thesis in Applied Ethics. Linköping: Centre for Applied Ethics, Linköping University. Available at: http://www.diva-portal. org/smash/get/diva2:23919/FULLTEXT01.pdf. [Accessed 29th April 2016].

Kung, H. 2007. *Islam: Past, Present and Future.* Trans. Bowden, J. Oxford: Oneworld, 562.

Keyserlingk, E. W. 1993. Ethics Codes And Guidelines For Healthcare And Research: Can Respect For Autonomy Be A Multi-Cultural Principle. In: *Applied Ethics: A Reader.* Oxford: Blackwell, 319–415.

Larijani, B., Zahedi, F. and Malek-Afzali, H. 2005. Medical Ethics in the Islamic Republic of Iran. *Eastern Mediterranean Health Journal* 11(5–6), 1061–72.

Lewis, J. 2003. Design Issues. In: Lewis, J. and Ritchie, J. (eds.). *Qualitative Research Practice: A Guide for Social Science Students and Researchers.* London: Sage Publications, 56.

Lurie, P. and Wolfe, S. M. 1997. Unethical Trials of Interventions to Reduce Perinatal Transmission of the Human Immunodeficiency Virus in Developing Countries. *N Engl J Med* 337, 853–5.

Macklin, R. 1999. *Against Relativism: Cultural Diversity and the Search for Ethical Universals in Medicine.* New York: Oxford University Press.

Mir-Hosseini, Z., Al-Sharmani, M. and Rumminger J. (eds.). 2015. *Men In Charge?: Rethinking Authority in Muslim Legal Tradition.* London: One World Publications.

Nanji, A. 1993. *Islamic Ethics.* In: Singer, P. (ed.). *A Companion to Ethics.* Oxford: Blackwell, 106–18.

Nuffield Council on Bioethics. 2002. *The Ethics of Research Related to Healthcare in Developing Countries.* London: Nuffield Council on Bioethics. Available at:

http://www.nuffieldbioethics.org/research-developing-countries/research-developing-countries-chapter-downloads. [Accessed 20th June 2015].

Oguz, N. Y. 2003. Research Ethics Committees in Developing Countries and Informed Consent: With Special Reference to Turkey. *Journal of Laboratory and Clinical Medicine* 141(5), 292–6.

Padela, A. I. and Punekar, I. R. A. 2009. Emergency Medical Practice: Advancing Cultural Competence and Reducing Healthcare Disparities. *Academic Emergency Medicine* 16(1), 69–75.

Ramadan, T. 2009. *Radical Reform: Islamic Ethics and Liberation.* Oxford: Oxford University Press, 207–32.

Rathor, M. Y., *et al.* 2011. The Principle of Autonomy as Related to Personal Decision-Making Concerning Health and Research from an "Islamic Viewpoint." *Journal of the Islamic Medical Association of North America* 43(1), 27–34.

Ryan, M. A. 2004. Beyond a Western Bioethics? *Theological Studies* 65(1), 158–77.

Sachedina, A. 2009. *Islamic Biomedical Ethics: Principles and Application.* Oxford: Oxford University Press.

Sachedina, A. and Ainuddin, N. 2004. *Islamic Biomedical Ethics: Issues and Resources.* Islamabad: COMSTECH.

*Sahih Bukahri, Book 18, Hadith 1750:* "Abu Hurairah (May Allah be pleased with him) said: 'The Messenger of Allah said, "It is not lawful for a woman to observe an optional Saum (fast) without the permission of her husband when he is at home. Nor should she allow anyone to enter his house without his permission." [Al-Bukhari and Muslim]. Available at: http://sunnah.com/riya-dussaliheen/18/240. [Accessed 29th February 2016].

Schulman, K. A. 2009. Ethical and Scientific Implications of the Globalization of Clinical Research. *The New England Journal of Medicine* 360(8), 816–23.

Shabana, A. 2013. Religious and Cultural Legitimacy of Bioethics: Lessons from Islamic Bioethics. *Medicine, Health Care and Philosophy,* 16(4), 671–7.

Sleem, H., El-Kamary, S. S. and Silverman, H. J. 2010. Identifying Structures, Processes, Resources and Needs of Research Ethics Committees in Egypt. *BMC Medical Ethics,* 11, 12.

Suleman, M. 2015a. Contributions and Ambiguities in Islamic Research Ethics and Research Conducted in Muslim Contexts: I — A Thematic Review of the Literature. Accepted by the *Istanbul Journal of Health and Culture* [In press].

Suleman, M. 2015b. Contributions and Ambiguities in Islamic Research Ethics and Research Conducted in Muslim Contexts: II — A Review of the Research Ethics Guidelines in 57 OIC Countries. Accepted by the *Istanbul Journal of Health and Culture* [In press].

Suleman, M. 2016. Does Islam Influence Biomedical Research Ethics? DPhil thesis. Oxford: University of Oxford.

ten Have, H. and Gordijn, B. 2011. Travelling Bioethics. *Medicine, Health Care and Philosophy* 14(1), 1–3.

*The Holy Qur'an.* Chapter 16, verse 97 "Whoever does righteousness, whether male or female, while he is a believer — We will surely cause him to live a good life, and We will surely give them their reward [in the Hereafter] according to the best of what they used to do." Available at: http://corpus.quran.com/translation.jsp?chapter=16&verse=97. [Accessed 27th January 2014].

*The Holy Qur'an.* Chapter 4, Verse 34. "Men are the protectors and maintainers of women, because Allah has given the one more (strength) than the other, and because they support them from their means." Available at: http://corpus.quran.com/translation.jsp?chapter=4&verse=34, [Accessed 27th January 2014].

*The Holy Qur'an.* Chapter 3, verse 104. "And let there be [arising] from you a nation inviting to [all that is] good, enjoining what is right and forbidding what is wrong, and those will be the successful." Available at: http://corpus.quran.com/translation.jsp?chapter=3&verse=104. [Accessed 28th December 2015].

Von Denffer, A. 1983. *Ulum al Qur'an.* Markfield, UK: The Islamic Foundation, 41–2.

Weindling, P. 2008. The Nazi Medical Experiments. In: Emanuel, E., Grady, C., Crouch, R., Lie, R., Miller, F. and Wendler, D. (eds.). *The Oxford Textbook of Clinical Research Ethics.* New York: Oxford University Press, 18–30.

Zahedi, F. and Larijani, B. 2008. National Bioethical Legislation and Guidelines for Biomedical Research in the Islamic Republic Of Iran. *Bulletin of the World Health Organization* 86(8), 630–4.

# CHAPTER ELEVEN

## Challenges in Islamic Bioethics

### *Khalid Alali, Gamal Serour, Alireza Bagheri*

### Summary

Bioethical dilemmas and challenges in Islamic countries vary significantly, and different topics receive different amount of attention by the academics, public, governments as well as media.

With advances in scientific knowledge, there are many emerging challenges in bioethics particularly in Islamic societies that are committed to faith-based solutions for those dilemmas.

The concept of Islamic bioethics is contested, and there is controversy how to characterize Islamic bioethics. By examining the concept and methodology of Islamic bioethics, this chapter presents several challenges in developing Islamic bioethics, such as the issue of principlism in Islamic bioethics; the relationship between ethics, law, and *fatwa*; the lack of public awareness and participation; as well as human rights in Islamic bioethics.

## Introduction

Ethics is an indispensable part of Islamic teachings, however, contemporary bioethics in the Muslim world is a relatively new field of inquiry. There are attempts to define bioethics, its concepts, and methodology in the Islamic context (Bagheri 2011), a task that is not without challenge.

Islam is a religion of ease (*yusr*) and not hardship (*usr*) and is directed to the benefit of humanity (2:185). In Islamic societies, the teachings of Islam have shaped Muslims' personal and social life as well as their practice and attitude towards health, illness, life, death, and the environment. These teachings are the main source for responding to ethical questions arising in biomedicine and healthcare decision-making. Islamic *Shari'a* governs the private lives of individual Muslims as well as public policies. In medical practices and services, healthcare providers and patients alike need to be reassured that these practices do not conflict with *Shari'a* to avoid situations of conscientious objection, and to ensure concordance with treatment (Serour 2014). However, Islamic rules and regulations are originally expressed as general principles and norms which are not expounded in detail and in many cases without textual ordinances offering explicit guidance; thus falling within the domain of juristic discretion (*ijtihad*). To respond to the ethical dilemmas raised by new advances in science and technology, Muslim scholars utilize the authentic sources of Islamic *Shari'a* to find applicable answers to those questions and queries. In order to provide ethical guidelines for such complex dilemmas in light of religious tradition, there is an ongoing constructive collaboration between Islamic jurists, as the experts of the Texts, and scientists, as the experts of the Context (Bagheri 2014).

Bioethical dilemmas and challenges in Islamic countries vary significantly, and different topics receive different amounts of attention from the public, governments, as well as media. An international study published in 2014 listed the top 10 bioethical issues in Muslim countries. The first challenge was the relationship between law, ethics, and *fatwa* followed by health resource allocation; human rights; bioethics capacity-building (education/training); patients' rights; brain death and organ transplantation; individual autonomy; Islamic principles of bioethics; abortion; and, finally, bioethics committees as number 10 in the list (Bagheri 2014). There are several major challenges in Islamic bioethics which influence the approach taken when dealing with bioethical issues. The importance of defining Islamic bioethics has been emphasized in the bioethics literature (Serour 1994; Sachedina 2009; Bagheri 2014). Elaborating on bioethical challenges in Islamic societies is instrumental in the efforts to determine the concept of "Islamic bioethics." This chapter examines challenges in Islamic bioethics and ethical dilemmas in Islamic societies.

## Islamic Bioethics: Concept and Methodology

The concept of Islamic bioethics is contested, and there is controversy over how to characterize Islamic bioethics. For instance should Islamic bioethics be based on principlism as in many western countries? If not, what are other options? Several scholars have been trying to define Islamic bioethics, its concept and methodology. It has been argued that "ethical judgments in Islam are an amalgam of the empirical — the relative cultural elements derived from the particular experience of Muslims living in a specific place and time — and the *a priori* — the timeless universal norms derived from the scriptural sources" (Sachedina 2009, 27). However, there is a fairly broad consensus that Islamic bioethics is in fact a series of Islamic perspectives on bioethical dilemmas, and Islamic jurists decide about the ethical evaluation of an act in specific circumstances and guide others by declaring it as necessary (*wajib*); prohibited (*haram*); permitted (*mubah*); recommended (*mustahabb*); or reprehensible (*mak'ruh*). In this sense, the role of juridical decision-making is to balance and correlate between divine command and human good.

Several Muslim bioethicists have stated that Islamic bioethics upholds the four principles of biomedical ethics proposed by Beauchamp and Childress in the West (Serour 2014; Chamsi-Pasha and Albar 2013). In comparing western and Islamic bioethics, Chamsi-Pasha and Albar (2013), argue that one can easily find all these universal [four] principles in the Holy Qur'an and *Sunna*. These scholars however conclude that the distinction between Islamic medical ethics and principlism-based medical ethics lies in the underlying religious basis of morality. However, Sachedina (2009, 8), emphasizes that "in Islamic bioethics, praxis precedes [the] search for principles and rules and customarily, when faced with a moral dilemma deliberations are geared toward a satisfactory resolution ... and justifications are based on practical consequences, regardless of applicable principles" (Sachedina 2009, 8, 27).

It should be noted that a search of bioethics literature reveals that many papers on Islamic bioethics have only searched for the Islamic equivalents of the four principles introduced by Beauchamp and Childress in their book, *Principles of Biomedical Ethics*.

If secular western bioethics can be described as rights-based, that is, with a strong emphasis on individual rights, then Islamic bioethics is described as being based on duties, obligations, rights, and virtues (Shad 1981). Islamic bioethics presents the ethical doctrine that supports the legal tradition in Islam; in other words it presents Islamic perspectives on bioethical issues. The scope of Islamic legal studies includes medical jurisprudence, but does not deal with biomedical ethics based on the current definition of bioethics. Sachedina, however, warns that the total absence of any discussion about the moral underpinnings of religious duties in Islamic jurisprudence renders bioethics beyond the scope of *Shari'a* studies. It is for this reason that in teaching Islamic bioethics we need to constantly avoid reducing the inquiry to *fatwa* investigation. Sachedina concludes that it is important to distinguish between a "legal-religious ruling" and an "ethical resolution" (Sachedina 2011). However, as observed by Farhat Moazam, discussions and rulings in Islamic bioethics are not fashioned in a vacuum but shaped by the interplay of perceived boundaries of authority within political and legal systems and existing societal norms (Moazam 2011).

Defining Islamic bioethics itself seems challenging and in need of the conjoint multidisciplinary efforts of the primary authority of Islamic scholars and physicians and bio-scientists with the lived experience.

## Challenges in Islamic Bioethics

With vast developments in scientific knowledge, research, and medical services, there are many emerging challenges in bioethics particularly in Islamic societies that are committed to faith-based solutions for those dilemmas.

### The relationship between ethics, law, and fatwa

In all religious or non-religious bioethics systems, the relationship between ethics and law needs to be discussed and defined. However, when it comes to Islam, another factor, namely Islamic juridical ruling or *fatwa*, plays a great role. In Islamic jurisprudence, ethical values are integral to the prescriptive guidance of the community. No legal decisions are made without a meticulous analysis of the various factors that determine the rightness or the wrongness of a case under consideration (Sachedina 2009, 7). As mentioned above, based on an international study among Muslim scholars, the relation between law, ethics, and *fatwa* was ranked as the number one priority among the top 10 bioethical challenges in Islamic countries. In Muslim societies, being bound to Islamic jurisprudence, it is important to first define the position of Islamic *Shari'a* on the questions raised by an ethical dilemma (Mohaghegh Damad 2010). In practice, the priority of the religious position is evident by the fact that scientists and physicians considering the application of a new biotechnology are keen to begin with an exploration of the opinion of Islamic scholars (*faqih*) on the biotechnology to ascertain if there might be questions of permission or prohibition. In Islamic societies, juridical opinions are compiled to document the responses by the various scholars representing different schools of thought to bioethical issues.

It should be noted that, in Muslim societies, the ethico-theological discourse is overshadowed by juridical rulings. As Sachedina argues, "although Islamic juridical methodology was firmly founded on some moral principles like rejection of harm and promotion of public good in deriving solutions that Muslims encountered in their everyday life, gradually, the judicial opinions were formulated without any reference to ethical dimensions of the cases under consideration." He further observes: "in general, ethical inquiry connected with moral epistemology or moral ontology is underdeveloped in the Muslim seminarian curriculum which is, in large measure, legal-oriented" (Sachedina 2009, 10, 19). Therefore, the relationship between ethics, law, and Islamic jurisprudence remains a challenge in Islamic bioethics, an issue that needs to be elaborated.

## The issue of principlism in Islamic bioethics

The question whether Islamic bioethics is a principle-based bioethics has become an important question in the related literatures. Several authors have tried to answer this question in the light of the four principles of bioethics proposed by Beauchamp and Childress. However, among the four principles of bioethics, autonomy has caused the most controversy not only in Islamic bioethics but also globally. For instance, it has been argued that in Islamic communitarian ethics, autonomy is far from being recognized as one of the major bioethical principles (Sachedina 2012).

On the other hand, Serour (1994) examines that, although the principle of autonomy is recognized in Islamic bioethics, yet when it contradicts public interest, precedence is given to the latter. Chamsi-Pasha and Albar also suggest that Islamic ethics upholds the four principles of biomedical ethics proposed in the West. However, they argue that the western attitude of individualism is not accepted as a basis in bioethics decision-making in many societies, and there are different cultures such as Muslim societies that do not give priority to autonomy as it is understood in the West. In fact, in Islamic jurisprudence axioms, avoiding harm takes precedence over doing good (Chamsi-Pasha and Albar 2013).

Among Islamic bioethicists there is a great tendency to elaborate on the principles of biomedical ethics based on Islamic teachings. So far, several Islamic principles have been proposed to deal with ethical issues. Principles such as the sanctity of human life (*ihsan*); public interest (*maslaha*); no harm no harassment (*la dharar wa la dherar*); necessity (*dharura*); and no hardship (*la haradj*). (Serour 2014; Chamsi-Pasha and Albar 2013; Larijani and Zahedi 2008).

Nevertheless, to emphasize the importance of ethical principles, Sachedina (2012), argues that "the principles and rules function as a bridge between revealed text and reason, correlating the conclusion as a normatively validated resolution. Islamic ethics requires the principles to be extracted from normative sources recognized by the community as 'Islamic,' and justification and legitimization are dependent upon moral principles and rules established in Islamic legal theory."

### Diversity among Islamic jurisprudence

With the advancement of science and technology, new issues are bound to arise which are not already addressed by the Islamic *Shari'a* outlined more than 1,400 years ago. Driving ethical principles for such emerging practices and research can be accommodated by *Shari'a* as long as they are intended to benefit humanity. Islamic countries are similar in terms of religious background, however, in Islam there is no central authority as in the Catholic religion. Therefore, due to different jurisprudence, diversity exists among them especially in dealing with newly emerging issues.

In Islamic bioethics, it is very important to define the position of Islamic *Shari'a* in dealing with a newly emerging ethical dilemma. In practice, if there are any ethical concerns in the application of a new bio-technology, scientists and physicians first seek the opinion of Islamic scholars (*faqih*) on the issue. However, in the absence of a central authority for all schools of thought in Islam, determination of valid religious practice is left to the opinion of qualified scholars of Islamic *Shari'a* (*faqih*). Accordingly, in dealing with bioethical questions in Islamic jurisprudence, if there is no textual ordinance (*nass*) offering explicit guidance on the issue under consideration, decisions on the matters fall in the domain of juristic discretion. It has been argued that in Islamic bioethics, discussions and rulings are not fashioned in a vacuum but shaped by the interplay of perceived boundaries of authority within political and legal systems and existing societal norms (Moazam 2011). However, given the fact that there are different schools of thought in Islam, the resulting rulings may differ based on juristic discretions. Such diversity exists even within each school of thought because of differing opinions among Islamic jurists. In this regard, different rulings between *Shi'ite* and *Sunni* are notable on such topics as surrogate motherhood, birth control, and assisted reproductive technologies among different Islamic jurists. In these cases, although the underlying principles are the same, the conclusions and rulings might be in opposite directions. For instance, there are opposite rulings about surrogate motherhood from prohibition to permission. This situation poses a challenge in Islamic bioethics.

### *Bioethics teaching and curricula in medical schools*

A bioethics curriculum has not been included in the curricula of medical schools in a large number of Muslim countries. Furthermore postgraduate bioethics courses have been scarce in most Muslim countries apart from a limited number of bioethics workshops organized by the World Health Organization's East Mediterranean Regional Office (WHO–EMRO) as well as UNESCO. In a large number of Muslim countries, this has resulted in the general lack of bioethics knowledge and its application in healthcare service and research. It is only relatively recently that a number of medical schools in Muslim countries have started to include bioethics in their curricula. Not only should bioethics be included in the curricula of all medical schools, but it should also be included in postgraduate courses and training programs in these countries. Another issue worth mentioning is that even where there are medical ethics courses, the curriculum is not based on "Islamic" bioethics. However, the assumption among healthcare professionals and institutions that the solutions offered to moral dilemmas in the western setting apply across other cultures is no longer valid.

That Islamic bioethics is not discussed in medical schools may arise from two factors: the lack of a well-defined Islamic bioethics approach as well as from the incorrect assumption that the solutions offered to resolve moral dilemmas in western settings apply equally well across other cultures. This challenge can be overcome by — among other things — including the methodology of moral reasoning in Islamic ethics in the medical curriculum. However, a close collaboration of bioethicists, Islamic scholars, and experts in medical education is needed to develop a comprehensive Islamic bioethics curriculum.

### The lack of public awareness and participation

In bioethical discourse, individual needs as well as larger societal concerns are considered in the decision-making process. However, there is a lack of public discourse in bioethics which poses a serious challenge to the development of bioethics in Islamic societies. Although several conferences and seminars have been run throughout the years, bioethics discussions do not include the public and decisions are not made by public participation.

In some Islamic countries, the lack of active national bioethics institutions such as national bioethics committees to lead national discussions and to guide the public as well healthcare providers can be an obstacle in bringing bioethics into the public sphere. Establishing such active committees in Muslim countries would provide ethics guidance and help in raising awareness about contemporary bioethical issues. These bioethics committees can cover all aspects of the field including education, research, as well as policy-making. Enhancing public discussion and involvement in bioethical topics and decision-making will bring a better public awareness and participation.

## Multiculturalism and global awareness about Islamic bioethics

Due to globalization, healthcare providers and patients alike move fluidly around the world. In multicultural societies, it is common for healthcare providers to provide medical services to patients with many different cultural and religious backgrounds. In the era of globalisation, multiculturalism has become a distinctive characteristic of many societies worldwide. Currently, the Muslim population consists of almost one-fourth of the world's population, and there are many Muslims living in non-Muslim communities and countries. Therefore, it is important for healthcare providers worldwide to understand not only their own traditions and values, but also those of the different cultural and religious traditions within their communities (Serour 2015).

Solutions to moral dilemmas in medicine based on the western traditions should not be presumed to apply across other cultures. As argued by Alastair Campbell (1999), global bioethics must respect the whole diversity of worldviews of ethics, both religious and non-religious. In practice, the lack of sufficient knowledge about the principles underpinning Islam's bioethical framework causes the delivery of culturally insensitive healthcare (Mustafa 2014). Currently, it is a challenge for Muslims who live in non-Muslim countries to have their ethical issues resolved according to Islamic recommendations. It is equally challenging for healthcare providers in the West to deliver culturally sensitive healthcare services to their Muslim patients.

Providing quality healthcare services which are culturally sensitive and ethically sound to Muslim patients requires healthcare institutions and healthcare providers to be aware of these religious and culturally sensitive solutions in medical practice and research. In reality, Muslim bioethicists generally are far more aware of western bioethics than their western counterparts are aware about Islamic ethics. It remains a challenge for Muslim scholars to explain Islamic bioethics to their non-Muslim colleagues and to provide insight into Islamic medical ethics, and thus enable non-Muslim healthcare providers to have a more productive discussion with Muslim patients.

## Misunderstandings about some Islamic traditions and rules

There are misunderstandings about some Islamic rituals and rules not only in the global bioethics community but also in some Islamic societies. For instance, female genitalia mutilation, which is not recommended in Islam, has been falsely linked to Islam on the basis of an unauthenticated *hadith*. In fact, medical research has clearly shown that this practice is associated with health risks and increased morbidity and even mortality, and has no benefit whatsoever (Serour 2010). If one applies the principles of Islam and other divine religions of not inflicting harm on human beings, this practice should be prohibited and even criminalized (Serour 2001; 2013).

There is also misunderstanding about human reproduction in Islam. The importance of marriage, family formation, and procreation has been highly emphasized in Islam. (Serour 2002; 2015). Islam also affirms the importance of purity of genes and lineages. As the Qur'an reads, "nor did he make your adopted sons, your actual sons" (33:4). However, some publications imply that Islamic bioethics is against contraception and family planning and supports unlimited procreation; and consequently it is unethical for Muslims to practice family planning (Serour 2013).

This view is based on an incorrect interpretation of the Holy Qur'an and *Sunna*. The consensus of juridical opinion in the Islamic world today is that family planning and contraception are to be encouraged as necessary to maintain a high standard of health for both mothers and children. Islam is a religion which encourages planning all aspects of life, including reproduction. Family planning was practiced by the companions of the Prophet Muhammad, who used *coitus interruptus*, and he did not forbid his companions from doing so (Gad El Hak 1992).

By analogy, which is one of the secondary sources of extracting Islamic laws, current temporary methods of contraception would be similar to *coitus interruptus*, which was used by the companions of the Prophet. Furthermore, Islam encouraged lactation for infants until two years of age which itself is a fairly effective method of contraception. It should be remembered that in Islam there is the principle of "necessity permits the forbidden," as it relates to human health. While sterilization as a form of permanent contraception is primarily forbidden in Islam, sterilization is allowed for specific health indications such as uncontrolled diabetes, heart disease, or congenital abnormalities incompatible with life. In such cases, patients may be sterilized after they have given their free, informed consent (Serour 2001).

Another misunderstanding arises with Assisted Reproductive Technology (ART) which was introduced around 30 years ago. Some commentators have claimed that ART violates Islamic bioethics because it allows scientists to handle human gametes and embryos and interferes with God's will. For Muslims, if ART is indicated by physicians as necessary for a married couple, it is permitted and even encouraged because it preserves humankind (Serour 2002; 2008; 2015). However, the *fatwas* among *Sunni* Muslims emphasize the necessity of maintaining purity of lineage. Thus sperm donations, egg donations, or embryo donations are not permitted. While most *Sunni* scholars would not approve surrogacy, a *fatwa* by *Shi'a* scholars has opened the door to third-party donation and, therefore, egg and sperm donation and surrogacy have gained acceptance among *Shi'ite* Muslims (Inhorn *et al.* 2010; Serour 2008). However, it might not be surprising to see a *Sunni* Muslim couple seeking egg or sperm donation based on his/her conscience. Alternatively a *Shi'ite* couple may hesitate to practice egg or sperm donation based on his/her conscience.

### Human rights in Islamic bioethics

The interconnection of bioethics and human rights is evident in several international bioethics documents such as the *Universal Declaration of Bioethics and Human Rights* (UNESCO 2005).

However, there are some concerns and reservations in Islamic countries regarding the human rights perspective. For instance, several Islamic countries did not sign the 1948 *Universal Declaration of Human Rights* because they were not satisfied the document was compatible with Islamic *Shari'a*. Later, in 1990, this concern was addressed by the Organization for Islamic Cooperation which developed the *Cairo Declaration on*

*Human Rights in Islam.* The Cairo Declaration referred to *Shari'a* as its "only source of reference" (Cairo Declaration 1990). However, the Cairo Declaration has been criticized because it refers to "Islamic *Shari'a*," a concept which lacks consensus, and about which there is diversity of opinion in Islamic countries (Kayaoglu 2013). However, Muslim scholars, physicians, and bioethicists alike seldom cite either of these human rights documents in bioethical deliberations. As observed by Turan Kayaoglu (2013), a significant obstacle to the promotion of the *Universal Declaration of Human Rights* in the Muslim world is the concern about its compatibility with Islamic *Shari'a*. He suggests that, from an international human rights perspective, the controversial nature of the Cairo Declaration lies in its claim of adherence to Islamic law. In the context of bioethics and human rights, if one references Islamic *Shari'a* to restrict the application of human rights, this shows how challenging it is to address and satisfy international human rights criteria in an Islamic context and *vice versa*.

## Conclusion

In Islamic societies, the teachings of Islam have shaped Muslims' personal and social life as well as their healthcare decision-making. In Islamic bioethics, it is very important to define the position of Islamic *Shari'a* in dealing with ethical dilemmas. In global bioethics as well as among Islamic scholars, there is a great attention to the concept of Islamic bioethics and its methodology in resolving bioethical problems. In determining the concept of Islamic bioethics it is important to identify and to address bioethical challenges in Islamic societies. This will bring a better understanding of Islamic bioethics in a global context. Finally, there is a demand to establish academic bioethics centers to promote Islamic bioethics in the Islamic world. Such bioethics centers can provide consultation, policy development, training, capacity building, and raising awareness among the public.

## References

Bagheri, A. 2011. Islamic Bioethics (editorial). *Asian Bioethics Review* 3(4), 313–5.
Bagheri, A. 2014. Priority Setting in Islamic Bioethics: Top 10 Bioethical Challenges in Islamic Countries. *Asian Bioethics Review* 6(4): 391–401.

Beauchamp, T. L. and Childress, J. F. 2013. Principles of Biomedical Ethics. 7th ed. New York: Oxford University Press.

Campbell, A. V. 1999. Global Bioethics: Dream or Nightmare? *Bioethics* 13(3/4), 183–90.

Chamsi-Pasha, H. and Albar, M. A. 2013. Western and Islamic Bioethics: How Close is the Gap? *Avicenna Journal of Medicine* 3(1), 8–14.

Gad El Hak, A. G. E. 1992. *Islamic Shari'a and Medical Issues in Gynecology and Reproductive Health.* Cairo: International Islamic Center for Population Studies and Research, Al-Azhar University. [Arabic and English].

Inhorn, M. C., Patrizio, P. and Serour, G. I. 2010. Third-Party Reproductive Assistance Around the Mediterranean: Comparing Sunni Egypt, Catholic Italy and Multisectarian Lebanon. *Reproductive BioMedicine Online* 21(7), 848–53.

Kayaoglu, T. 2013. *A Right Agenda for the Muslim World? The Organization of Islamic Cooperation's Evolving Human Rights Framework.* Analysis Paper No. 6. Doha: Brookings Doha Center.

Larijani, B. and Zahed, F. 2008. Islamic Principles and Decision Making in Bioethics. *Nature Genetics* 40(2), 123.

Moazam, F. 2011. Sharia Law and Organ Transplantation: Through the Lens of Muslim Jurists. *Asian Bioethics Review* 3(4), 316–32.

Mustafa, Y. 2014. Islam and the Four Principles of Medical Ethics. *Journal of Medical Ethics* 40, 479–83.

Pellegrino, E., Mazzarella, P. and Corsi, P. (eds.). 1992. *Transcultural Dimensions in Medical Ethics.* Frederick, MD: University Publishing Group, 13.

Sachedina, A. 2009. *Islamic Biomedical Ethics, Principles and Application.* New York: Oxford University Press.

Sachedina, A. 2012. Defining the Pedagogical Parameters of Islamic Bioethics. *Iranian Journal of Medical Ethics* 1(1), 34–42.

Serour, G. I. 1992. *Ethical Guidelines for Human Reproduction Research in the Muslim World.* Cairo: International Islamic Center for Population Studies and Research, Al-Azhar University.

Serour, G. I. 1994. Islam and the Four Principles. In: Gillon, R. (ed.). *Principles of Healthcare Ethics.* London: John Wiley and Sons, 75–91.

Serour, G. I. 2001. An Enlightening Guide to the Health-Care Needs of Muslims. *Lancet* 358, 14.

Serour, G. I. 2008. Islamic Perspectives in Human Reproduction. *Reprod Biomed Online*; 17(Suppl 3), 34–8. See also Serour, G. I. 2013. Ethical Issues in

Human Reproduction: Islamic Perspectives. *Gynecological Endocrinolology,* 29(11), 949–52.

Serour, G. I. 2010. The Issue of Reunfibulation. *International Journal of Gynaecology & Obstetrics* 109(2), 93–6. See also Serour, G. I. and Ragab, A. 2013. *Female Circumcision: Between the Incorrect Use of Science and the Misunderstood Doctrine.* 2nd ed. Cairo: International Islamic Center for Population Studies and Research, Al-Azhar University and UNICEF Egypt.

Serour, G. I. 2015. What Is It to Practice Good Medical Ethics? A Muslim Perspective. *Journal of Medical Ethics* 41, 121–4.

Shad, A. R. 1981. *The Rights of Allah and Human Rights.* Lahore: Kazi Publications.

The Organization of the Islamic Cooperation. 1990. *Cairo Declaration on Human Rights in Islam.* Available at: http://www.oic-oci.org/english/article/human. htm. [Accessed 15th December 2015].

The United Nations Educational, Scientific and Cultural Organization (UNESCO). 2005. *Universal Declaration on Bioethics and Human Rights.* Paris: UNESCO.

# Index

# About the Editors

**Alireza Bagheri-chimeh**, MD, PhD, is assistant professor of medicine and medical ethics, in School of Medicine, Tehran University of Medical Sciences, Iran and a research affiliate, Centre for Health Care Ethics, Lakehead University, Canada. He is a member of the UNESCO International Bioethics Committee (IBC) and an elected fellow of The Hastings Center (USA). Dr. Bagheri is a member of the High Council of Organ Transplantation and a member of the ethics committee of the Middle East Society for Organ Transplantation. He is also a senior editor of the *Encyclopedia of Islamic Bioethics* and a member of Editorial Board of the *Encyclopedia of Global Bioethics* and serves as the editor of the *Intercultural Dialogue in Bioethics* book series. Dr. Bagheri was a clinical ethics fellow at the Joint Center for Bioethics, University of Toronto, Canada (2006–7), Erasmus Mundus visiting professor, University of Leuven, Belgium (2007–8), an Edmund Pellegrino fellow and a visiting scholar in the Center for Clinical Bioethics in Georgetown University, USA (2007–09). He has edited several books including, *Medical Futility* (2013), *Biomedical Ethics in Iran* (2014) and *Global Bioethics* (2016).

**Khalid Abdulla Alali**, PhD, is the associate vice president for academic affairs and an associate professor of human genetics at Qatar University, where he previously served in several leading positions such as the

251

director of the foundation program, vice dean of the College of Science and the head of Health Sciences Department in the College of Arts and Sciences. Dr. Alali was the chairperson and a member of the World Commission on the Ethics of Science Knowledge and Technology (COMEST) in UNESCO. He is currently a member of the Arab Committee for Science and Biotechnology Ethics and chairs Qatar University's and Qatar Biomedical Research Institute's IRB committees. He is also a member in the IRB committee of Weill Cornell Medicine-Qatar, Sidra Hospital and Qatar Bio bank. Dr. Alali also established the first Cytogenetic Laboratory at Hamad Medical Corporation in Qatar and has several publications to his name in the fields of cytogenetics and bioethics especially in relation to the Arab and Islamic world.

Printed in the United States
By Bookmasters